Big Me, Little Me:

A Survival Guide for Littles by Littles

By: Penny Berry

Dedications

To My Daddy:

For whom this book would not be possible without.
To be your Little is the greatest feeling in the world.
Mahal Kita!

To My Bubby:

For whom it is a joy to spend my life with.

To Every Little:

Embrace who you are from the inside out.
You are special, unique and a ray of sunshine.
Never stop dancing through life.
Thank you for your support and Happy Reading!

Table of Contents

Introduction:

H i there! If you're reading this introduction, I applaud you. Normally when I pick up a book I skip the introduction. Or I begin reading it, and if the words capture my eye then I usually purchase the book outright. I look to see if the author is speaking to me because I want to feel a connection. That's why we read books, right? We yearn to learn from one another. This book is me, a Little, talking to you. Yes, you. It's just you and I now. So, let's take some time and chat together.

Odds are if you picked up this book you're a Little... or a Mommy or Daddy. Maybe you're new to the world of DDLG/LB and are curious about it. Or maybe you're looking for that Little to love and dote on. I get it. I was there, too, a few years ago. I didn't know the terminology. A Dom came into my life like a tornado and opened my eyes to a part of me that was always there... and yet, it was never tapped into until that moment. It forever changed me, and I know if this path is for you... it will change you too. Don't be afraid, my friend. I'm here to break everything down into bite-sized pieces and make the journey much easier. Let's start with the basics:

What is age regression and what is the difference between age regression and little space?

Age regression is an umbrella term meaning anyone of any age who reverts (or mentally slips) into a mindset that is younger than their biological age. You can be a 50-year-old who mentally wants to act like a 20-year-old. Or a 20-year-old who wants to be a 5-year-old. The possibilities are as unique as the individual. Little Space is a term used among littles as the mental place you shift into to get into the little mindset. It is also used in speech when speaking to members of the DDLG/LB community to describe when they are in a little mindset. For example, you might hear: "I went into little space, and Daddy and I had a playdate at the playground!". This means the little got into a frame of mind, where they regressed in age and during the duration of the date... they were in a little headspace! See? Piece of cake!

Now there are things you'll read or hear about that are quite negative myths and stereotypes when it comes to DDLG/LB. I want to knock these out of the way here in the introduction. Why? Because I don't want the book to be filled with negativity. I want to clear your mind of any misconceptions right off the bat, and then fill it with rainbows, happy thoughts, and excitement! (Or, at least I'll do my best!). So, let's clean house of this negativity, shall we?

Chapter I.

A Glimpse into the DDLG Community

Myth #1: Littles are only females.

This is incorrect. There are plenty of little boys out there who are wonderful, littles too! Hence why I respectively use DDLG/LB to stand for Daddy-Dom Little Girl/ Little Boy. Although I should also note that there are also plenty of wonderful mommies too! So, if you want to be super technical and correct it would be DDMD LG/LB. Now, everyone is included. :)

Myth #2: Why would an adult be attracted to an adult with a childlike mindset?

Let's look at it another way. Everyone in the world has natural talents and gifts, yes? You do too! Some people are excellent public speakers. There are people who are charismatic. Other people are natural nurturers. It comes to their natural ability to love, care, and cherish for others. They have an innate ability to connect with people who need healing, or love, or simply to be heard in a way that requires compassion and humility. Mommies and Daddies are some of the gentlest people you'll ever meet. They understand that a little is someone who requires patience, time, and understanding. They get joy from helping others. To see a biological adult act like a child is simply a person reaching out their arms for a hug. The dominant is more than willing to step into those arms to hug them back. They also are very flexible by nature. Here is a little who wants to get down on the floor and color because it makes them happy. So, the caregiver gets down on the floor and colors, not because it does something for them, but because it brings joy to the little. It nourishes them, and in turn, seeing the little happy makes the caregiver happy. It's pure, selfless love.

Myth #3: Daddies and Mommies are Pedophiles.

This is perhaps the most angering, and upsetting myth surrounding the DDLG/LB community. There is a stark difference between pedophiles and caregivers. Let me explain in very blunt words here. There are laws for a reason. Any responsible daddy, mommy, or little will tell you that the laws of the land should *always* be obeyed. Children are defined as people under the legal age of adulthood (18 and younger). DDLG/LB is not meant for them. Daddies and Mommies **are not** attracted to children! They are attracted to the *joy and love* of caring for another **legal adult** who regresses to a younger age. I would bet that 99% of everything out on the internet that says otherwise and mentions pedophilia is written by an ignorant person looking to spread hate. Our community is filled with like-minded adults in consensual, mature, loving relationships.

Myth #4: All Mommies and Daddies Are Very Sexual (aka Tinder Daddies)

I heard a statement recently that really summed up sex well. I'll paraphrase it here. What you do with your sex life, is up to you. It's your consent. It's your body. When you enter into a binding relationship within the D/s (Dominant-Submissive) world, you have a contract. There is something written down somewhere that shares your core values, limits, rules, etc. I'm married to my Daddy and even I have a contract! It's because you value and love yourself enough to always have limits in place. You also need to know the limits and expectations of your caregiver. That said, there are plenty of DDLG/LB relationships that do not include sex of any kind! Are there daddies and mommies out there looking to get their freak on with littles? Sure. There are players even outside of the DDLG community. It's no difference, really. But this small fraction of the population cannot define the larger, more-encompassing community that actually has true, binding relationships.

Myth #5: All Littles Are Sexual in Little Space

Again, it's your body, your choice, and quite frankly... it's your own private business what you do (or don't) in the bedroom! If you are in little space and that carries over to the bedroom... you do you. If you're a proud little who doesn't have sex in little space... that's fine too! I've seen one too many arguments within the DDLG/LB community where people argue online about if this lifestyle is a kink or not, or if sex in little space is normal or not. Honestly, it's silly to argue about such things. The only way you will know if a Little wants to have sex in little space is to ask. And if you feel comfortable asking, go for it. Otherwise, just keep those curious thoughts in the back of your mind.

Myth #6: DDLG is gender, race, and age specific.

This is obviously false but I'll dissect it anyway. As you'll read further in this book, there are a ton of littles from every race, age, and walk of life. I would love to meet an older (50+) little one day. One day that will be me! Who knows? Maybe I'll be paving the way for "little grandma's!" Ha! No, but in all seriousness, you can be any age, weight, race, sexual orientation, gender, etc. and be a little or a caregiver. We don't judge around here! :)

Myth #7: DDLG is a kink.

In order to have this stereotype you first need to know what the definition of a kink is. A kink is defined as, a sexual taste or preference for a person. This assumes that a person gets sexually aroused at the idea of an adult in little space. Perhaps this is the case. For other littles and their caregivers, they simply enjoy the act of being in little space together and it does not include sex. So, is DDLG a kink? If your personal tastes are attracted to it, and you gain sexual arousal from being in little space, then yes, it's a kink. There's absolutely nothing wrong with that. And if you aren't sexually aroused by things in little space, but instead you simply enjoy being a little and/or caring for one, then no, it's not a kink. That's perfectly great too. There isn't a right or wrong here. It's all about personal preference.

Myth #8: Littles are underage.

I'll keep this answer here short and sweet because in a few pages you will read my full opinion and stance on underage littles. Here is the gist of it and I daresay the vast majority of the DDLG community's opinion as well: No, littles are not underage. Why? Because that, my friend, would be against the law. Littles are legal adults in consensual relationships that may or may not include sexual activity. They are not underage minors!

Now that we have cleared all of that negativity.... let's focus on something happier! Talking to your little is a very rewarding activity for any caregiver. For the sake of this book, I'm going to use the pronoun "we" to refer to us, the little community. That will help you to (hopefully) see deeper into our mindset. When we go into little space, mentally we begin to shift. The stress of the day melts away. We don't think of our jobs, bills, or anything in our adult lifestyle. As such, we often take on the tone and behavior of the age we regress to. This can also include a change in how we speak.

Every little has their own tone and speech pattern. Sometimes the letter "w" gets substituted into words more often. (For example: "widdle" means "little" or "verwee" means "very"). Other times littles will give nicknames for ordinary items or their favorite foods. As you develop a deeper relationship with your little you will learn all the little terms they enjoy. Here are a few commonly used ones:

- **Ageplay**- An umbrella term for two consenting adults who engage in role play where one adult regresses to a different age.
- **Daddy Dom/ Mommy Domme**- a commonly used term for a dominant who is a daddy or mommy.
- **Caregivers**- a non-gender specific term used for an adult who helps care for a little.
- **Little Space**- the mental space in which a Little slips into to embody being a little. Also used to describe the duration of time in which a submissive is in a little headspace.
- **Littles**- the term used for a submissive who identifies as a little and regresses to an elementary school age (or younger).
- **Middles**- the term used for a submissive who age regresses to age around middle or high school age.
- **"AB's"** - an abbreviation for Adult Baby, or an adult who regresses in age to embody the mind and behavior of an infant.
- **Sippy**- a nickname for a sippy/drinking cup.
- **Baba**- a nickname for a baby bottle.
- **Binkie/Binky/Paci**- a nickname for a pacifier
- **Nappy**- a nickname for a diaper (UK origin)
- **Wawaa**- a nickname for water
- **Blankie/Woobie**- a nickname for a comfort blanket to sleep with
- **Plushie/Stuffie**- a nickname for a plush/ stuffed animal
- **Hungie**- a word meaning to be hungry
- **Jammies**- a nickname for pajamas
- **"Play time"/ Boomies**- a nickname for sexual intercourse
- **Tushie**- a nickname for bottom, butt, rump, etc.
- **Princess Parts/ Private Parts**- a nickname used in little space to talk about genitalia
- **Tinkle/ Potty**- a term used to alert the need to use the restroom/washroom

The Issue of Underage Littles and Caregivers:

I saved this chapter as the last part of the introduction because it can be quite controversial among the community. The opinion expressed below is purely mine. Please use your own judgment and act accordingly.

I have seen some very heated discussions on websites, YouTube, and Instagram on the topic of underage littles and caregivers. Now I want to explain in detail why I feel the way I do. The role of a caregiver/ dominant is a serious one. Not only does the dominant play with toys, listen for hours as the little babbles and confides their innermost feelings, but they also are tasked with the responsibility of guiding their little. They are the anchor in their life. They are there to mentor, be a mature voice in times of strife and confusion, and be a rock for the little to lean on. All of these things require maturity, life experience, and tons of patience.

Likewise, the dominant is looking for certain things from their little to create a healthy bond. The little has to be able to identify and articulate their feelings so that the dominant can guide them. They have to have the wisdom to understand the difference of when "bratting" is okay, and when they have gone too far. (Don't worry, we'll get into that more later). But in short, the little has to also have life experience to understand what is uplifting to the dominant and be able to meet their needs as well. A Daddy/Mommy- Little relationship is one of power exchange. As such, it takes two mature, legal adults to create a consensual bond for that to happen.

So, can a little or caregiver be underage? If you want my opinion... no. I don't think they can. Can you be curious and read all about it? Absolutely! Go for it. Can you attend events to begin to get a feel for what it takes to be in the BDSM/DDLG community? Of course! However, given that this community does have sexual themes and individuals who do view it as a kink, I tend to err on the side of caution (and the law) and suggest that you wait to be 18 to fully enter the community as a little or dom. That protects you and your partner. Trust me, it's cleaner on all sides and you gain life experience in the meantime.

Chapter II.

The Psychological Side of "Little Me"

I think you're more of a submissive than you realize.

I remember when my first Dom said those words to me. I was stunned. My brain was spinning thinking, "I'm sorry. What? I'm a what?". Admittedly, at the time I was a bit "vanilla". People in the BDSM community use the affectionate term for people not into the kink scene. Being very curious by nature I began googling the term and pouring through hundreds of websites. Everything I read intrigued me. I began to identify with certain parts of the terms described. I like to be happy and free yet I like to serve and take care of others. I like to have someone in my life to lean on and to guide me. I'm not the best with rules and can be a bit stubborn. I knew that I needed to head to the bookstore and do some deeper research.

As my first dom-sub relationship ended I felt like a piece of debris floating in the ocean. I was lost. A part of me had been opened up in the hours of conversations and confiding pieces of me that I hadn't told anyone... ever! I had begun to accept that I was a submissive, but I wasn't quite sure how to proceed without a dom in my life. I needed something more concrete. Unlike many, I *do* like labels. They give my brain a sense of reasoning. I ordered, Elizabeth Cramer's "*Submissive Training Manuals*" (both volume 1 and 2) and devoured them as if I were reading the Bible. She took the confusion that I had, and began to make sense of it. There were labels out there in the BDSM community with various groups of people. I just needed to find my tribe.

Being a little isn't the easiest thing to embrace. How do you explain to people that you enjoy Disney movies just as much as a kid? Or that you secretly want the My Little Pony pajamas instead of the women's ones? How do you convey that when you're upset you want to curl up into a ball and be soothed instead of sitting down and talking "like a mature adult"? There are questions, intense feelings, and a path of discovery and self-reflection that each little goes on. Your path is yours alone, but know that every little goes on relatively the same road.

As you begin to embrace that you are, in fact, a little you'll see that it's not something that you choose to become. It's something that you already are. Now you just have a term for it. If you go explore sites on the web (as listed in later chapters) you'll also find that there are a lot of people out there who are just like you! Now, how cool is that! Yes, we exist and many are "out and proud" of their Little status. There are local meet-ups and large conventions that cater to Littles with or without a caregiver. There is a community of us here to support and welcome you with open arms and lots of snacks! But before you dive into a pile of plushies, it's important to know if you truly identify as a Little or if you are just curious about us.

Being little is a part of who you are. You can't turn it off, but you can suppress it. (As you'll learn about distinguishing between "Big Me" and "Little Me"). Maybe you've always felt like a child at heart. You smile and are drawn to things designed for children. The way your brain is hardwired, you naturally think in terms that adults might deem as "immature" or "selfish". You're not immature nor are you selfish. You are an adult who has an inner little waiting to be loved, guided, nurtured, and be able to be given permission to express yourself to the world.

Society has stigmas about people who like things deemed for childish. They have sayings such as, "act your age" or "grow up!". But you aren't going to find those in the DDLG community. Instead you will find peace, acceptance, and a community of people who embrace differences and similarities. So, I encourage you to accept that part of yourself. Love who you are and let that part shine.

Triggers That Make You Feel Little Are Normal:

I'm one of those "hippie dippy" people who believe in surrounding yourself with items that make you happy. This includes items that are designed to help you get into little space. There will be times that you will be out in public and you'll see something that makes you slip into feeling little. This is entirely normal and nothing to be ashamed about. Little space should be a mental place of retreat where you are your happiest, unencumbered, and freest sense of self. It's a place where you can release the adult side of you and embrace everything that makes you happy. I encourage you to take time to make a list of things that you enjoyed as a child. What did you want to be when you grew up? What are dreams that you had? What are toys that you enjoyed as a child? You can get those items and surround yourself with things that trigger you into that warm, fuzzy state of mind.

As you become more comfortable with being little you will see the pure joy of being in that head space and how valuable it is to your mental health. I'll elaborate. Did you know that infants are burped by their parents because gas can be painful? As we get older we're expected to deal with this same discomfort on our own. But, when you're in little space, one of the greatest joys is simply being burped. Imagine for a moment, snuggling up to your caregiver. You're in their arms, so you're safe and protected. You feel warm, and their natural scent is inviting. After having a sippy of your favorite beverage, they hold you in their arms and gently rub and pat your back. For several minutes, maybe even a half of an hour, you lay there against their body just being soothed of potential gas. You burp adorably so. There isn't any shame in passing gas or burping because to them they are soothing you of any pain, and to you there is relief and comfort. Everyone is happy and fulfilled. It's an incredible bonding experience. The trigger becomes that every time you see your favorite beverage you can smile and yearn to be burped afterward. This is the power of items used in little space.

Recognizing Your Feelings in Little Space and Helping Out Your Dom/Domme:

Every little is guilty of not fully expressing their feelings at some point or another to their Dominant. It's part of the process of bonding with your caregiver. We lean on them so much that we expect them to be mind readers. Wouldn't that be nice! But sadly, they can't be. No one can be. Being an adult, little is highly complex. On one hand you project this image of innocence and juvenile behavior, yet you are still biologically an adult with complex thoughts and emotions. There must be balance between the two. To achieve this, I suggest coming up with a system with your Dom that allows the two of you to connect and discuss feelings. For example: if you're feeling little and need to go into little space you can use a code word. This signals to your dom that you need time to mentally release. Likewise, if there are adult issues and emotions happening, it's probably best to not be little when you discuss things of that nature. Can you imagine talking about bills in little space?

Daddy: Angel, did you pay the water bill?

Angel: Nope!

Daddy: And why not?

Angel: Because it's stupid!

That wouldn't work so well! Feelings happen. Intense feelings bubble up, and it's important to tell your caregiver how you're feeling both in and out of little space. Sometimes it's necessary to take a "time out" and say that you need to be "Big Me" for a moment to air your feelings. Other times littles won't want to talk about their feelings. They will go little, but usually those feelings come out in other ways. They become snappy, feisty, and overall just plain grumpy! Then the Dom has to figure out what's going on and begin to dissect the root of the issue. It's far better to come clean to save time, emotion, and strain on everyone.

Using Little Space to Help Soothe Mental Illnesses:

I'm quite passionate about mental health because only in the past decade has society begun to be more receptive towards "hidden illnesses". That said, if you are struggling with a mental health issue I want you to know something first and foremost: **It is never your fault that you are struggling this way!** Let me say that again. The feelings you have, the thoughts you wrestle with, the behavior you may exhibit, and the obstacles you deal with... are NOT your fault! Just as people have physical illnesses and need to see a doctor, so too do people with mental illnesses. There is no shame in seeking out a doctor for help. You never, ever need to feel badly for having an illness of any kind. These are professionals who have dedicated their life towards helping people feel better and get well again.

I'm not a mental health professional, so in addition to whatever outside healthcare you seek, I am simply here to discuss the power of using little space to ease symptoms of depression and anxiety. Little space is a sacred head space. There is a reason that we all have an inner child. The brain naturally wants to protect itself. That's why we have a "fight or flight" area of the brain designed to detect danger and respond accordingly. Our inner child is that mental place where all things are possible. It's a place where the world so scary, where we don't have Trump as president, and people aren't hurt. It's a place of optimism and hope. It's also a powerful place to disconnect from everyday intrusive thoughts that are common among individuals with depression and anxiety.

Depression and anxiety often get clumped together in the mental health field, but they are quite different. Both make a person feel isolated, but in different ways. Depression (especially chronic depression) makes the world feel gray. A person slowly loses that sense of hope and wonder. Let me make it clear: no one wants to have depression! I have never met a person who *wants* to be depressed. It is a chemical imbalance in the brain that makes a person feel that way. This can be difficult not only for the person suffering from depression but for those around them. Littles who have depression can struggle to find their self-worth. Their Dom will probably have to work a little bit harder to find things that connect on a deep level with their submissive. But if you can find that one plush toy, or a tea set, a video game, a physical place that brings back good memories, then you have a spark to get the kindling going for little space. You just need a hook that the little can grasp onto to begin to shift their mindset. Little space can alleviate the feelings of isolation, lethargy, sorrow, and loss of appetite by tackling them one by one. In little space the dom/domme is right there on the floor playing with you so you aren't isolated.

The little might feel fatigued or lethargic. This is a common symptom with depression. The caregiver can hold their little and rock them lovingly for hours if need be. When feelings of sorrow arise, allow your little to cry. Reassure them that everything is okay, and that you are there, and will continue to be there for as long as it takes and then some. Lastly, the loss of appetite is another common symptom with depression. It might take time and lots of coaxing, but in little space many littles use food as a tool to help get into a happy, mental headspace. You'll see dino nuggets or smiley french fries eaten. Lots of littles have favorite snacks such as: goldfish, cookies, cheerios, and cheese cubes. Getting a bit of nourishment into your little when their appetite is down will also make them feel better. (Tip: greens are an excellent tool for fighting depression and pack a powerful, nutritional punch. So, try creating a platter of their favorite fruits and greens like broccoli with dipping sauce!).

Anxiety is a whole different "beast". Unlike depression that leaves a person feeling in a slump, anxiety has the opposite effect. A person becomes hyper-vigilant and overly cautious to the point where the fear can be crippling. Intrusive thoughts become commonplace and can scare a person with anxiety so much that they refuse to do anything at all. Did you know that after embracing someone for 2 minutes straight, the entire nervous system relaxes? When was the last time you hugged someone for two consecutive minutes? The power of physical touch has a profound effect on someone with anxiety. People with anxiety often: feel jittery, sweat, have panic attacks with triggers, suffer from intrusive thoughts, feel restless, overthink things, and generally worry much more. Little space can help soothe some of these symptoms. In little space, the submissive is encouraged to mentally let go. For a sufferer of anxiety, this can be difficult but not impossible. I would encourage the caregiver to give their little items that naturally comfort them: a favorite storybook being read to them, a plushie or blankie, food that makes them happy, and tons of snuggle time.

Part of being in little space is being with your daddy or mommy often. You naturally want to snuggle and be loved on. As negative, intrusive thoughts come and go, your little can have a code word or a system with you (the caregiver) to help ease through each one. Little space becomes a coping mechanism. For example: your little crawls into your lap to play. You're snuggling and loving on them. They're smiling and all is well. Then suddenly they mumble a few words to you to signal that a fear is creeping up in their mind. Like any thought that every person has, we acknowledge that it is there, and then we release it. For a person with anxiety, they simply need help in releasing the thought from their mind. So, you snuggle them a bit closer. Softly, together you begin to sing:

Bad thoughts, bad thoughts go away.
Good thoughts, good thoughts here to stay.

Maybe you sing the song, "Favorite Things" from the "Sound of Music". As you're singing they begin to imagine: raindrops on roses, whiskers on kittens, bright copper kettles, and warm, woolen mittens! This imagery begins to shift their mental focus. Or you sing another happy song that distracts their brain until the fear has passed. Your little is relaxed again and then little space can continue.

I want to take a moment to talk about panic attacks. A panic attack is completely different from simply being afraid of something. When you get scared you might startle or gasp aloud. For a moment your body enters shock, but it quickly recedes as the source is identified and you respond to the situation. A panic attack can occur at any time, any place, and for no apparent reason. For many, it can feel and mimic the symptoms of a heart attack. You begin to sweat, struggle to breathe, and feel dizzy. Your systems go into overdrive and it can feel difficult to think straight. The panic attack can last minutes, or up to several hours! It's terribly difficult for the person affected. When your little is having a panic attack you, the caregiver, will most likely not be able to use verbal commands to help them cope. However, you can be instrumental in helping them come down from the attack faster and easier with your actions.

I recommend first making sure your little is in a safe place. If you're out in public try identifying what could be the source of the attack. Are you in a crowded place? Is the noise level too loud? Is it too hot? Is your little dehydrated? Try and find the source and remove it as quickly as possible. If possible, get your little to a new, calm, safe environment to begin relaxing. The "come down" from a panic attack can leave your little one tired, vulnerable, and sad. This is natural because their entire body went into overdrive to fight the fear. Be patient and hold them close. They simply need to know you're there and that they aren't alone. Mental health can be a beast to tackle, but I firmly believe that little space and the tools used with littles can be invaluable to adding a bit of happiness, love, warmth, and joy back into a person's life.

Why "Bratting" Isn't Encouraged:

What is "bratting" and why isn't it encouraged? Why does any little brat? Let's examine the question more bluntly. Why do children act out? There are many reasons: they want attention, they're having a rough day, they have something to say but can't find the words to get it out, etc. Similarly, littles brat their caregivers for the very same reasons. However, the dynamic between a parent and child, versus a dominant and little is quite different. As a parent you understand that your child is your responsibility. You signed up for all of the tantrums, crying, snotty noses, and ear-piercing moments the minute you gave birth. As a dominant, you have patience, yes, but at the end of the day it is still two consensual adults. In other words, a little knows better than to act out like that! Still, we do it for the variety of reasons (and more) stated above.

So, what makes it so toxic to a relationship? Dominants are attracted to littles because of the core similar traits they exhibit. Littles are kind, loving, happy individuals. They are people pleasers and gain great joy from doing a task right for their dom. They enjoy a myriad of things, but they often love to share those hobbies with the ones they are closest to. Daddies and mommies gain such pleasure from being around their littles because they are positive people. When a little "brats" they shift the dynamic a bit. In the power exchange, the little is forcing the dom to dig deeper and be more patient to get their little to be happier, soothed, and back to their emotional baseline. Now, every now and then if a Little acts out and brats, okay, it happens. But on a regular basis? Let me be blunt: would *you* want to deal with a bratty person day in and day out? Of course not. While it can be "fun" to do that while in little space, it's best to check yourself before you emotionally hurt your dom/domme and use a better form of communication instead. I suggest drawing, writing letters to your dom/domme, or snuggling up and just talking! If it's something very personal and you feel the need to brat, don't. Go out of little space and just talk about it. Trust me. It keeps everyone much happier.

The Importance of Your Little Name:

William Shakespeare once said, "a rose by any other name would smell just as sweet" ... well, that may be so, but you can't have just *any* little name. It doesn't work that way. Entering into little space is much like a performer walking on stage. You become the persona that you wish to project. You suspend your mind and dive into a world of imagination. It's a happy place filled with laughter, plushies, cuddles, and everything bright and beautiful. It's a place where innocence takes the forefront and you can leave your cares behind. It's a magical land made just for you and your dominant. When you enter little space you also leave behind your "real" identity. You embody a new name, your little name, and that name holds great power to you. Over time you might, (as I have), prefer to be called by your little name. But just any submissive name won't do. I could never be called Angel or Princess. Those are far too fluffy names for me, but perhaps they hold special meaning for you. Here are a few examples of submissive names to help you get into little space:

- angel
- baby doll
- baby girl
- beautiful
- boo
- cookie
- cupcake
- cutie/ cutie pie
- doodlebug
- dumpling
- gorgeous
- honey bun
- kiddo
- kitten
- little girl
- little boy
- little one
- love
- pancake
- peanut

- pet
- petal
- poppit
- princess
- prince
- precious
- snickerdoodle
- sugar
- sunshine
- sweetie

So, you can see that the list of names is vast. Above is only a small fraction of the possibilities. What matters is finding *your* identity so you can fall into little space easily. Are you a sweet, little princess? Or are you a gentle petal? Only you know what name feels right. When you hear your dom say that name... you'll just know. Bear in mind that just as people change, so too will your D/s relationship change and evolve over time. That's perfectly natural.

When my Daddy and I first came together he gave me the name Mouse. He wanted me to understand the full meaning of being small, quiet, obedient, and still. He wanted to take my bouncy, happy-go-lucky personality and reel it in so that he could train me to be the submissive that he desired me to be. It was difficult at first. I didn't like the name Mouse. But, I listened to him and soon realized that perhaps I needed to learn to be quiet. He taught me how to meditate and relax more. Over several months of training we bonded more deeply than I ever could have imagined. I sat on a plush floor cushion by his side, quiet, just enjoying holding space with him. Finally, Christmas time came and he surprised me with a small ceremony to mark the next chapter of our relationship... and he gave me my new (and final) name: kitten! I was so touched and felt happily in love with him.

So, when picking your name choose something that matters. Let your dominant guide you to a name that works for both of you. Enjoy being called by your new name. Think of it as your "secret identity". That name is your happy place. It's a small, sacred place in your life where you can be your most authentic self. Dance, laugh, play, and become who you were meant to be... a little!

Finding a Safe Caregiver: What to Look For & Signs or "Red Flags" to Avoid:

You now have some idea of a name you want. Or maybe you don't have a little name at all! That's perfectly fine. A name will come when the time is right. It's difficult to 100% feel sure about your little name when you don't have a dominant to guide you. However, the good news is that there are *many* daddies and mommies out there yearning to care and love on a little just like you! Yes, YOU! Y-O-U! You are special, beautiful, unique, and different and that is what they are looking for. Despite popular media suggestions, daddies and mommies don't care if you're tall, short, large, skinny, or any other color of the rainbow! They yearn for a little who is kind, obedient, loving, happy-go-lucky, funny, and someone who is eager to please. They long for someone who is emotionally sure in themselves, yet who wants to open up to them too. They wish for someone who is ready to give over power and compassion, yet still retain their own opinions too. Remember: being a submissive *does not* mean you're a doormat! Far from it, actually.

So now that you're ready to find your mommy or daddy, let's talk about what to look for in a healthy caregiver. Close your eyes for a moment. No, wait. Don't close your eyes because then you can't read this book. Okay, let's envision a high school cafeteria. I know, we were all there once. I'm sorry. But, imagine yourself in a cafeteria full of people around your age. You are looking sharp in your best outfit! I mean, you are working it today, girl! Your hair in on point! People are eyeing you up and down as you march with utter confidence into the room like you own the place. This is the secret power that you now hold when finding a dom. You aren't scrambling and begging for someone to collar you. No way, honey! You are scoping *them* out to see who is good enough for you! You have standards, and selection processes that would put the TSA to shame! You eye over potential matches with a scrutinizing (but not condescending) look. You're here for a serious, long-term relationship. Not just any mommy or daddy will do. They need to be in it for the long haul too. So, what are you looking for?

Like any healthy relationship you want someone who is:

- **Emotionally grounded:** They need to be able to control their emotions without freaking out. Violence among littles is completely unacceptable.
- **Clear in Communication:** They need to be able to give clear, concise directions so that they can guide you without you feeling like you don't quite understand what they mean. Miscommunication is the bane of many arguments.
- **Exude Confidence:** They are a dom for a reason, right? They need to project that they have it all together and they can lead you through life. If they come across as timid, or mumble all the time, then that isn't going to make you feel dominated.
- **Patience:** let's get very real here for a moment. Littles (like any child) can push every button that a dominant has. We just do. We don't necessarily mean to. But it happens. Daddies and mommies have to have the patience of gods to deal with us…. which is why we love to serve and love on them loads too. Wink, wink!
- **Know What They Want:** Not every D/s relationship is the same. Some couples are live-in, while others are long-distance, and others are completely online. When you enter into a relationship with your dom they need to be able to state exactly what they are looking for in the relationship, (and you do too!). This will help create a strong foundation for you both.
- **Be Kind:** This might seem obvious but you'd be surprised at how many people out there forget to be kind to one another. Your dom should be kind, loving, warm, and understanding. This relationship is special for you both, and little space should be a place where there isn't a *need* to argue or bicker.

Okay, so we have some qualities above for you to start screening potential dom/dommes. Now let's examine what we *don't* want in a caregiver! Not long ago someone told me about a "Tinder Daddy" experience they had. Y'all, I didn't even know that was a thing! So, of course I had to look into it and it turned out to be a (thankfully, small) group of people who use tinder to… you guessed it… hook up with littles posing as a daddy. Um, no. Can I just rant here for a moment? Bear with me. As a little you open yourself up emotionally and physically. We yearn for someone to love on us, guide us, and make us feel small. We allow ourselves to become vulnerable and timid. Why in the world would we want someone who is only in it for the hook up?! Gross! I get that we look 100% hot AF in a onesie, but c'mon...

Now back to other red flags to look for in doms/dommes. Let's take a mental journey together into "Bad Date Land". In Bad Date Land, every dom/domme is the absolute worst-case scenario that you could possibly find. Every date leaves you questioning if there are good daddies and mommies out there at all! (Spoiler: there are tons). But, let's focus on all of these dominants who are displaying classic "red flags" and what you should avoid at all cost:

- **Too Much, Too Fast:** This dominant asks you for pictures within hours of meeting you. You might feel a bit taken aback. Share pictures of yourself to a stranger this soon? Trust your gut. If the dom is ready to get to know you, then why give them your identity so soon? Let the mystery linger and feel them out for as long as you feel comfortable. If he's asking for pics. (or nude pics!) then hit the road, Jack...

- **The Shark:** Did you know that sharks can smell blood in the ocean from miles away? Just like a shark, there are doms who smell out submissives new to the BDSM scene. They target submissives who know very little about the lifestyle because they feel that they will obey them more. Knowledge is power, and these dominants don't want you to have any. If you meet a dominant who doesn't want anything to do with you because you know a thing or two about what you want as a little... then just say buh-bye!

- **Mr. Condescending:** There are a ton of ways to communicate with your little besides being a jerk. Nothing gets me fired up more than someone talking down to me. I don't know about you, but if you want me to obey, then just ask nicely. Right? If you're acting all high and mighty, or you treat me like I'm dumb, not only will I not feel little, but I'll get so angry that you can be sure that I won't be with you. Steer clear of these types too.

- **Mr. Keep-You-In-A-Box:** This is a dangerous type of dom/domme. Remember how I said, "knowledge is power"? This type of dom doesn't want you to have any. The Little community is vast and colorful. There are conventions held throughout the year all over the world and plenty of online forums for you to connect to. (See Chapter 7 for resources). This dom doesn't want you to connect with other littles. They don't want you to read books on being a little, or take you to conventions to show you off on their arm. They want to keep you hidden away with little knowledge or connection to others. It's a means of control, and quite frankly, a healthy dom doesn't need to control you like that to get your attention. If you meet a dom/domme like that, run away fast.

- **The Explosive Type:** Just as you wouldn't flip out and scream at a child, a dom/domme should never lose their temper and scream at their little. In little space you are much more open emotionally. You are wearing your heart on your sleeve, but you can't if your dom can't control their temper. If you meet a dom who has a short fuse, walk away as quick as you can and save yourself a lot of heartache.

- **No Dotted Line:** A lot of people think that a D/s contract needs to be something formal, legal, and binding. It can be. But usually it's just a simple word document that both parties type up together that lists hard limits, rules to abide by, soft limits, and most importantly, safe words to be used to stop all play sessions. Remember: being a little is part of the BDSM umbrella. Meaning that many D/s couples also experiment with other kinks and fetishes while in little space as well. It's great to have a written contract to put everything out there for you and your caregiver to know and understand. If you meet a dom/domme who isn't willing to write a contract with you, then not only are they being unsafe, but they are neglecting to care for your safety as well. Find a safe word that resonates with you to use in play. Red means stop, now! Yellow means slow down, I need a moment. You get the idea. You need a dom/domme who *wants* to know these words to better care for your needs. Don't let some person say, "I'm your dom and therefore I know what your limits are". Nu uh, honey! Sign the dotted line or I'm out of here! You get the idea.

- **King of Everything:** So, you found a dom/domme that you're screening to be a potential match. That's good. But then you slowly figure out that they have rules for you. This isn't a deal-breaker... yet. Except that their rules are *a lot* of rules. They tell you what to eat, how to dress, and what to call them. Okay, that's not totally unusual. They tell you how to groom your pubic hair. Now we're charting into "red flag" territory. They tell you how to spend your free time, and what hobbies you should be doing. Now, we're out the door. Do you get the idea? There is a difference between having some basic rules that guide you into little space and make you feel little. This is uplifting. But if the dominant's rules restrict you to the point where you feel stifled then it isn't going to work. (This is another reason why a contract is so important). Talk it out with your dom and see if you can come to an agreement on the rules. If not, then turn on that cute heel of yours and sashay away!

- **Baby, Baby, Baby:** Now, us littles, love a good compliment or twelve, but if you're scoping out the dom's and you come across one that slides up to you saying: "hey there baby girl..." .... cringe. Cringe, hard. What makes you, Dom, think that you can call me your baby girl so soon? Yes, we love being flattered on, swooned over, and spoiled rotten. We are littles, duh! But, as I shared back in "Choosing a Little Name" chapter, a name is sacred ground. Don't let someone call you any name before the relationship is set. Otherwise he/she can "bye bye bye!".

- **Using the Relationship as a Means to Control:** Oh, this type of dom/domme triggers me so hard, so forgive me if I rant for a moment. There are dominant's out there who believe that it is perfectly acceptable to use communication (or withholding contact from you) as a means of punishment to the little. This is never... no, let me boldface this... **it is** <u>**never okay to use your D/s relationship as a means of punishment**</u>. Healthy dominants will have already read books on how to properly punish their little without breaking them down as a person and harming them emotionally. It's a fine balance between control and obedience. Withholding communication not only hinders the relationship because you cannot express your feelings to your dom, but it doesn't allow for conflict resolution. This type of dom wants absolute control and authority over you and doesn't value your opinion and feelings. Steer clear of such people.

- **Too Much Baggage:** It is the role of the dominant to lead and guide you to help you become your best self. It's a large task for anyone to take on, but dominants are special people who long to care for other people. Arguably they are the kindest, most generous people in the world. Having such a large responsibility means that they have to be grounded themselves. If you sense that a potential dom has their own baggage/ mental health issues, then they won't be able to guide you properly. There is nothing wrong with having mental health issues, but in a position with such power and responsibility, you need to have your life in order. It's like the airline announcement before takeoff: please take care of yourself before you try taking care of others. Make sure your future dom/domme is grounded and knows what they want from you before you relinquish control to them.

The 10 Commandments of Littles

When I was writing this book and I came to this chapter, I envisioned two giant stone tablets. Much like the biblical stone tablets these would be large for all to see. Except unlike the ancient texts, little commandments would be covered in glitters and painted in the brightest of colors. There would be stickers, glitter glue, and fluffy pom pom's adorned around the edges. It would be the cutest 10 commandments that ever existed. Now that you have the image in your mind, let's dive in:

Commandment I: Treat your mommy or daddy the way you want to be treated. Strive to be loving, respectful, and listen with an open mind and heart.

Commandment II.: Be honest with yourself and your caregiver about your feelings at all times.

Commandment III.: Love and accept every part of your Little self. You are uniquely beautiful.

Commandment IV.: Develop a trusting bond with your caregiver based upon two, consensual adults who share the same goal and vision: to be in a DDLG/LB relationship that is fulfilling and nurturing to both parties.

Commandment V.: Remember to have FUN! A huge part of the appeal for daddies and mommies is that Littles are people who know how to have a good time. So, smile, relax, and let your Little side shine!

Commandment VI.: Surround yourself with items that uplift you in Little Space. Whatever those items, plushies, toys, etc. may be, bring them into your space so that you feel naturally drawn to (and can relax in) little space.

Commandment VII.: Do not go out of your way to "brat" your caregiver. The grumpies happen. Bad days happen. But no one wants to deal with being manipulated. So be kind to your caregiver, and they should be kind to you too!

Commandment VIII.: Always have safe words in place for play sessions, little space, etc. They are vitally important to both you and your caregiver. This allows both parties to know if something needs to stop immediately. Likewise, you can have a designated word with your caregiver when you need to go into Little space and let your little side come out to play.

Commandment IX.: Discuss a suitable punishment with your caregiver while out of little space. Both parties should be mindful of any triggers that spanking, time out, etc. might cause.

Commandment X.: As you choose your caregiver and they choose you, it is critically important to know what you're seeking in a caregiver and to share what your needs are. For example: Are you an adult baby? Or are you a Little? Maybe you're a Middle?! Do you enjoy diapering as part of your little space routine? Or maybe your little space time is completely non-sexual? These are important things to share with your caregiver so you two can be on the same page at all times.

How to Separate "Big Me" and "Little Me":

It's inevitable as littles that there are times when we are in "big me" space and need or want to go little, or we are being little and then we have to shift into "big me" space again. It's just life. But before we break down the intricacies of both, let's examine what "big me" and "little me" is. "Big Me" is the normal, ordinary everyday adult you. It is the space that you embody when you aren't in your DDLG/LB role. For the sake of keeping things straight mentally, we affectionately call our adult selves "big me", and our inner little, "little me". "Big me" has to deal with bills. We have to pay the rent or mortgage. We have to take care of the kids. We have to deal with phone calls, emails, and courses at the university. We have to go to a job. "Big me" can easily get stressed and overwhelmed.

But "little me" is entirely different. It is the place that is quiet, and guarded from the world of prying eyes. It is the place where you can be silly, happy, and laugh often. It is the space where you can dress up in whatever makes you feel good simply because you want to! It is where those childhood dreams come to life again, and you find that age is simply a number suspended in time and space. It is a place where you can live and let live. Love without hesitation. You can be emotionally available and innocent. You can talk and take on the little you that has been there deep inside, just waiting to come out and play. It's the space where you don't need to feel silly or stupid for dressing in rainbow clothing. It's a place where you can color outside of the lines. It's that happy part of you that believes that anything is possible and that certain things are absolutely magical. It's a beautiful thing to be a little and I encourage you to embrace it fully.

You'll find in time as you go in and out of little space, that you will grow more comfortable with "little me". Your pattern of speech will change. The tone of your voice might become higher too. The many thoughts that come flooding your mind daily, will turn off while you're in little space and it will become a place of mental (and physical) refuge. But until you reach that point of understanding you might have some questions that arise in the process. Are you crazy or weird for wanting to wear diapers? Are you silly for wanting to have your own tea party with plushies and dolls? Is it strange that you feel most comfortable with a pacifier in your mouth? What will people think if they see that you have a baby bottle or a sippy cup?! All of these questions are normal, and are a part of the process of getting to know the little side of yourself.

As "big me" you are expected by society to act a certain way. There is a certain etiquette in the way you dress, and act, that should be adhered to. There are formalities in the way we speak and address others that is expected when you are "big me". In many ways, "big me" is restrained by societal pressures. While we could view this as a negative thing, the key is to find happiness and balance as both your adult and little self. Yes, you can't run around in diapers while out on public transit, but you can keep a small lovey-trinket in your pocket to feel as you're riding on the way to work. You might not be able to use your baby bottle on your lunch break at work, however there is nothing stopping you from getting an adorable water bottle to carry with you! Do you see my point? There are ways to be discreet in public and keep the little side with you while you're away from the privacy of your home.

Likewise, "little me" doesn't have much to worry about at all! Those pesky chores never get done in little space because what child wants to clean house?! No, little me is ready to play and never wants to go to bed at the end of the day. Like Peter Pan, "little me" never wants to grow up and wants to play until your muscles are spent and your skin was kissed by the sun. It's a beautiful thing, yes, but if you never went out of little space, nothing would ever get accomplished. It's a fine balance, my fellow littles. Learn to love both parts of yourself and you'll feel most at peace.

Littles and Parenthood: Is it possible to be both?

I have read many articles and books that state that littles absolutely, cannot become parents. I think there is a common misconception that if you're a little, you lack the maturity to also be a parent. But as I stated in the previous chapter, there is a time and place to enter little space. This goes hand in hand with parenthood. How do I know? Because I am a parent and a little as well! Now you might be thinking, how is that possible? Do my children know? How does that even work?! The short answer is: scheduling little time after their bed time. Now I'll give you the long answer.

Ask anyone who knows me intimately and they will tell you that when it comes to being a mother, I embody the true spirit of a mama bear. I am first and foremost always a parent first! I believe that when you choose to create life, and bring a child into the world that you have the emotional, moral, and physical responsibility to put them above anything else in your life. Period. That includes being a little. Your child needs you to be fully present in their lives and that means that your time gets divided. But you know what? That's okay! Embrace scheduling your day and you are sure to have plenty of little space time.

Now I want to dive a bit deeper in the aspect of being a little around children and should your child know about you being a little. When I first got into the BDSM lifestyle I heard a quote that really stuck with me: as a general rule of thumb, do not scare vanilla people. In other words, don't push your BDSM lifestyle onto people who aren't in it because then you're making them feel uncomfortable and that's unnecessary. So, too, do I believe that your little space should be a private place for you and your caregiver alone. Wait until the kids have gone to bed to then slip into little space so that your mind is relaxed and you're fully present in the moment. If you have older children and they are curious about you being a little, then it is at your discretion if you wish to disclose that information. But never forget to put being a parent and meeting their needs first, and above all else!

Sex in Little Space and Non-Sexual Littles:

Back in chapter one I discussed common myths and misconceptions about the DDLG/LB community. It is not pedophilia. Littles and their caregivers are two <u>consensual adults</u> who choose to enter an adult relationship that may, or may not be sexual in nature. For some reason the topic of sex within the DDLG/LB community brings about heated discussions. I'll give you the basic reason why the community often becomes divided on the issue.

The issue: DDLG/LB is a kink, which is under the BDSM umbrella, therefore sex is permissible and often encouraged between a little and their dom/domme. VS. a D/s relationship is not a kink, and is a part of the BDSM umbrella but is a power exchange between two adults and therefore it is up to the two parties to choose if sex is involved or not. Non-sexual littles are permissible.

If you're like me then you're probably thinking, "why does it matter what people do in the privacy of their homes?". In truth, it doesn't matter! But people love labels and DDLG is often demonized by arrogant people saying that dominants are pedophiles. So, the community gets "up in arms" about what should and should not be acceptable as a whole across the community. I know, it's silly. But let's examine this issue on a deeper level so we can see where the disconnect within the community stems from.

In my opinion, this entire debate arises from trying to understand the role of a Daddy or Mommy and their attraction to littles. Why would a grown adult want to be a mommy or daddy to a little? Are they attracted to the visual fantasy of a child? Or is it something different? These are common questions but without understanding, the dominant gets judged very harshly. Daddies and mommies are people who have a need to care for others. It isn't an act of arousal. That is something entirely different. They have an emotional need to care for their partner (in this case, a little) and to nurture them to the greatest of their ability. They seek to understand their little in the greatest capacity and to learn how their mind works. Much of the D/s relationship is all about domination of the mind, rather than the body. This is the same with a daddy/mommy and their little. The dominant learns what the little wants to get out of life, what goals they have, what weaknesses they are struggling with, and then they seek to create a path for them to learn to become better people to achieve their personal goals. If the little wants to lose weight to become healthier, the dominant will make rules for their little so that they can only eat healthy food and they must work out for 30 minutes a day. The little doesn't have a choice because it's a rule, but by doing so, the dom is paving a way for their little to reach their personal goals. The dom becomes fulfilled at seeing their little succeed with their help. It feels good to help others.

In terms of sex, entering into a sexual relationship is a serious matter regardless if the relationship is DDLG/LB or not. Sex is serious! It's an emotional act with many physical repercussions if not done safely. Often times there is confusion that daddies or mommies are sexually attracted to their little while in little space. If this is the case, and both you and your little agreed to sex while in a play session, do you. But it isn't fair to assume that every daddy or mommy and their little has sex in little space. Many, many couples go into little space for the enjoyment of simply being little. Littles get to play with their caregiver and have fun, while the dominant gets fulfilled by seeing their little so happy. All of the plushies, bottles, toys, etc. are simply props. At the end of the day, it's two adults having enjoyment together.

Sexual arousal is different. Many littles keep their sex life separate from their little space and that's perfectly fine. We can all agree that the DDLG/LB community is a branch beneath the BDSM community, but having sex with our dom is a personal choice. Having sex in little space is a choice. That's what the contract between the dom and submissive is for. (Do you see this recurring theme?).

So, too, is it an acceptable choice to have a DDLG/LB relationship that is completely non-sexual. There are just as many littles who have caregivers that do not engage in sex at all. You don't need to have sex to get into little space. Little space is a place for you to become little and take on the qualities and characteristics of your inner child. It is the place where you can color, dance, play with toys, watch animated movies, etc. and just relax. If sex isn't a part of that space, that's perfectly fine.

Key Points:
- DDLG/LB relationships are a part of the BDSM community
- Not every dom/domme finds sexual attraction in little space
- Not every little wants to have sex in little space
- If you do want sex in little space, put it in the contract between you and your dominant
- If you don't want sex in little space, make sure to put that in your contract too
- Whether you have sex in little space or not, there is nothing wrong with you. It's personal choice in which no one should judge you one way or another. We are one community. Let's support each other.

Chapter III.

What's In My Diaper Bag?: Tools For the New Adult Baby

*W*hat is an adult baby? Why would an adult be attracted to an adult baby, and what qualities do adult babies display? Imagine the most relaxing place in the world when you were a child. Where was it? Do you have your answer? Think way back as far as your memory can recover. That place was special. It was someplace warm and inviting. You felt at ease. You felt safe. Your needs were met and there was something magical about that little place that always stuck with you. This is the space in which the adult baby thrives. Adult babies are adults who enter little space around 0-3 years old. They yearn to be snuggled and loved upon. They love the comfort that a soft nappy and a gentle, cotton onesie provides. They are soothed by the touch of a soft, plushie and a pacifier in their mouth. Their bottle nurtures their need for a snack while they watch a program from their childhood that makes them feel happy.

The adult baby is keenly aware that it is a suspension of the imagination just like any other little within the DDLG/LB community but they are unique in the tools that they use to get into the little mindset. Adult babies often custom design furniture to create a crib or high chair for themselves. These tools are so helpful in making them feel more little. Just seeing their tiny nook makes them smile. Adult babies can range from those that are mostly non-verbal to those around aged 2 or 3 years, that use "baby babble" to indicate their needs to their dominant. The adult baby is special in that because their needs are so great, they can deeply fulfill daddies and mommies who wish to take care of them. The dom's cut up their food, rock them to sleep, or read them a book. They love being tucked into their crib, or to splash around in a bubble bath while being scrubbed down by their mommy or daddy.

The very mundane things in life suddenly become beautiful and playful with an adult baby. Folding the laundry can quickly turn into a game of peek-a-boo which leaves both the little and the caregiver laughing. The adult baby can make music, drumming with spoons and bowls, while the dom cleans up the dishes after snack time. The adult baby is a special type of little deserving of all the love, time, and attention that a dom can give. While the adult baby is only one of three major types of littles, it is one that dominant's find very rewarding to connect with because they can fulfill the nurturing need that they have.

Using the Menstrual Cycle As a Tool For Connecting In Little Space:

Being a little is difficult sometimes. Being an adult baby can be *very* difficult sometimes. There are times when you have a need to verbally express yourself but the words just won't come out right! Oh, the frustration of it all! This is especially the case right around the time when females are nearing their period. For 5-7 days we bleed, feel bloated, have mood swings, and generally feel fatigued. It can be downright awful and slam the brakes on wanting to go into little space.... or can it?

Writing and compiling this book has allowed me the luxury of being able to examine various types of littles and the nature of their relationships. Adult babies often have "lovie routines" or routines of personal hygiene that are an integral part of the relationship. This can include: diapering, powdering the private parts, rubbing lotion on the skin, bathing, brushing their teeth, etc. This got me thinking that having a dom nurture and love their little through the period cycle can be a powerful, and beautiful way to bond through a very natural part of life.

Think about it this way: for 5-7 days the little is going to be bleeding. If she is wearing her diaper/nappy, the blood will collect and pool there. This makes for easy clean up. If the dominant slips on a pair of disposable gloves and wipes their little down with diaper wipes, this is another way to love on their little. Most women feel disgusting and "heavy" during their period. But by having their dom love on them through their cycle there is a sense of compassion and acceptance in this time of vulnerability. It's telling the little that it's okay that she is bleeding. She can still be little no matter what state her body is in. It's not gross. There's nothing to be ashamed of. It's just blood. We all have it. It's a part of life. You clean it up, and toss the diaper in the bin. But using the adult baby's hygiene routine to connect on a deeper level like this can strengthen the bond between little and caregiver greatly by adopting this new practice.

Quick Tips & Tricks To Care For An Adult Baby:
- Warm up their baby blanket for 5 minutes in the dryer right before bed. A warm snuggle item will soothe them to sleep.
- Invest in a baby wipes warmer. They are inexpensive but will soothe your adult baby when you are doing a hygiene routine.
- Look for pieces of furniture that allow you both to sit and rock together. Amazon has some great love-seats that also rock back and forth. This can be a rewarding and meaningful spot to use in your home.
- 6 months + mason jar fast flow nipples are the best option for bottle-feeding. They will allow your adult baby the ability to drink without sucking too hard on the nipple and mason jars are very cheap and versatile to use in the home.
- Lastly, invest in adult onesies. They are one of the best clothing items to purchase for your adult baby that will get them into little space quickly.

15 Helpful Tools for New Adult Babies on Amazon:

As you begin your journey into creating a space for you to explore being an adult baby there are some inexpensive tools that can help you along your way. All of these products can be purchased off Amazon cheaply. I want to show you that you can create a fun, bright, engaging space to be an adult baby without breaking the bank! Now let's dive into these products:

1. Littleforbig Adult Bib, 2 pack- $12.99 USD
2. Littleforbig Adult Pacifier- $7.92 USD
3. Littleforbig Pastel Onesie- $19.99 USD
4. Littleforbig Adult Nursery Diapers- $33.24 USD
5. I <3 daddy onesie by Littleforbig- $25.80 USD
6. Mason Jar Nipple, Fast Flow 6+ Months- $9.99 USD
7. Foam Bath Letters and Numbers- $10.95 USD

8. Amazon Elements Baby Wipes, 480 count- $11.01 USD
9. Comfy Critters Stuffed Animal Blanket- $27.99 USD
10. Melissa & Doug Jumbo Coloring Pad- $4.99 USD
11. Schylling Tin Hot Air Balloon Mobile- $20.88 USD
12. Aveeno Baby Calming Comfort Lotion, Lavender & Vanilla Scent- $7.69 USD
13. 4 Pack Pokemon Socks- $12.90 USD
14. Baby GUND, My First Teddy Bear- $9.99 USD
15. Peppa Pig Toothbrush, Brush Buddies, 2 Pack- $3.96 USD

Things to Make Your Adult Baby Smile:

1. Create a diapering or personal hygiene routine and do it daily with them.

2. Make sure to incorporate story time regularly. (Head to the library together!)

3. Feed your AB their meal with children's utensils while they wear a bib. If you don't have a bib, don't stress! Tuck in a napkin around their neck and you're good to go!

4. Give your adult baby a bath, and gently wash them down with a soapy washcloth.

5. Try swaddling your AB in a cozy blanket. Did you know that there is a trend in Japan where people pay to be swaddled by professional swaddlers? It's true! Google it! It is wonderful to promote relaxation and relieve stress from the body.

6. Hug your adult baby for at least 2 minutes straight. Scientists have figured out that compassionate, physical touch that lasts for longer than 2 minutes, has proven to relax the central nervous system. It slows down your heart-rate and makes you feel at ease. Hooray for snuggling!

7. Place a night light next to your AB as they sleep to soothe them in their slumbers.

8. Bottle feed your little one regularly and don't forget to burp them afterward! I recommend mason jar fast-flow (6 month+) nipples.

Chapter IV.

Welcome to My Playpen: Tools for the School-Aged Little

*W*hat is an adult little? How are they different from an adult baby? Why would someone be attracted to an adult little? And what qualities and characteristics do adult littles display?

Unlike an adult baby that often uses a crib, an adult highchair, diapers, etc. to enhance time in little space, an adult little focuses more on regressing into a mental age space of age 2–8 years old. They are usually much more into toys, coloring, painting, singing, dancing, going to the playground, and watching animated movies with their caregiver. Adult littles make up a larger percentage of the DDLG/LB community as the activities and behavior within varies widely. Like adult babies, littles also enjoy being closely attached to their dominant. They, too, enjoy bottle feedings and sucking on a pacifier. They are usually sweet, loving submissives who crave pleasing their daddy or mommy by drawing pretty pictures, being silly, or snuggling up close.

Adult littles can also be broken down into a few generalized categories. There are littles who identify as "kittens" and enjoy being submissive to their master while incorporating some pet play into little space. Other littles identify as "lolitas" and draw inspiration from manga and the harajuku fashion movement. They dress in a lolita style that reflects frilly dresses with pastel colors. Still other littles enjoy wearing onesies much like adult babies! The names given to adult littles varies, and like any D/s relationship, the name given is unique between the bond of master and submissive.

The bond between a daddy/mommy and their little one is special and unique. Littles are submissives who relish slipping into a space where they can wear their emotions on their sleeve. Dominants of a little often find that they don't have to work hard at figuring out what their little is feeling, because their behavior displays the emotions. Unlike adults, when a little is happy they will sing, dance, laugh, smile, twirl, etc. Likewise, when a little is upset, the dominant must be extra patient and understanding as their submissive might throw a temper tantrum. Littles are often characterized as being "brats" to their dominant but not all littles enjoy bratting their caregiver.

Quick Tips & Tricks To Care For An Adult Little:
- Littles rejoice in having a caregiver who is gentle and compassionate. Remember to guide your Little, while still being kind and understanding.
- Coloring is one the best activities to do with an adult little. Not only is it therapeutic, but it helps keep the mind in little space.
- Bottle feeding is a wonderful activity to do with your little. I recommend purchasing a mason jar compatible fast-flow nipple (off Amazon) to create a simple, dishwasher friendly bottle. Then you and your little can snuggle up and you can bottle feed him/her while snuggled up. It's one of the best feelings in the world.
- When speaking to your little, your delivery of speech makes all the difference in the world if you two can enter little space. Try using gentle commands such as: "Daddy is going to order dinner for us now" or "Hold Mommy's hand as we cross the street" to help instantly shift your submissive into the little mindset.

- Lastly, most littles love everything pretty. Each little has their own style but all of us love gifts from our Dom/Domme. As such, a collar is an important gift that only our caregiver can give. It's a gift that is scared and should not be given lightly. It symbolizes the bond that you two hold together. Try surprising your Little with a collar that you think represents the love that you two hold together.

15 Helpful Tools For New Adult Littles On Amazon:

You've done a bit of soul-searching and decided to venture down the path of being a Little. Congratulations! The process of self-discovery in becoming a little is a special one. You'll find as you enter little space that it is like a breath of fresh air. It's a part of you that was always there, but it took a special moment to bring that piece of your soul out. Maybe you're bubbling with excitement and you've started Googling "DDLG" and finding all kinds of YouTube videos over the subject. There are many resources to read and it can be overwhelming. But in truth, it doesn't need to be.

Just as every child is different, so too is every little unique and special. The toys you connect with, and the activities you enjoy are exclusive to you. However, there are a few common items that you'll see many littles use to enhance their play space and help to keep the little mindset alive. They are as follows:

1. The First Years' Sippy Cups- $4.93 USD
2. Little Sleepy Heads Toddler Pillow, Elephant Print- $14.40 USD
3. Kirecoo Toddler Utensils- $10.99 USD
4. 5-piece Goodnight Moon Dishware Set- $15.54 USD
5. Goodnight Moon Book- $5.89 USD
6. Large Water Doodle Mat- $17.99 USD
7. John N. Hansen 1-50 dot-to-dot game- $5.75 USD
8. North States Superyard 8-panel Playard- $109.99 USD
9. Little Golden Books Set- $32.75 USD
10. Hugme Lace Lolita Bloomers- $16.99 USD
11. Papa Bear/ Daddy's Girl Bracelet Set- $16.99 USD
12. Riding Crop- $11.99 USD
13. Portable Time Out Mat- $15.82 USD
14. Record Your Voice Book, "All the Ways I Love You"- $32.69 USD
15. Daddy & Me Picture Frame- $9.85 USD

Things to Do to Make Your Little Smile:

1. Hold their hand when you're out and about

2. Be sure to cut up their food before serving it to them. (Bonus points if you put thefood on a pretty children's plate!)

3. Praise your little when they do a task right.

4. Take your hands and put your littles hands in yours and wash them together before meals.

5. Make sure to tuck in their plushies/ stuffies and kiss each one goodnight as you tuck your little into bed.

6. Make a "night cap" tradition by giving your little a sippy of their favorite beverage while you have a drink.

7. Burp your little after mealtimes by having them snuggle up on your lap and gently rubbing and patting their back.

Chapter V.

That's So Kawaii! Tools for the Adult Teen & Middle

hat is a Middle? What qualities or characteristics do Middles have? Is there a difference between a Middle and the "Naughty Schoolgirl" fantasy as depicted on many adult websites? In the world of DDLG, no group is more underrepresented and often overlooked then that of Middles. I want to be gentle, and move with great care as we dissect this subcategory of DDLG because Middles deserve their own praise and attention equal to adult babies and adult littles. So, what is a Middle? A Middle is a legal adult (and submissive) who regresses to the age of someone in early to mid-adolescence. Let's pause here for a moment and go back to our days as a teenager. Let's remember what things were like when we were an early teen. Our emotions were riding high. The world was our oyster. For some it might have been a time of rebellion. Teenagers experience highs and lows rapidly as hormones fluctuate and the body continues to grow. But this development period is a critical piece that paves the way for adulthood, because adolescence is the time for experimenting with your image.

One minute you feel like wearing all black and dressing "goth" and the next, you put pink stripes in your hair. One-minute JNCO jeans are a fad and you're wearing the baggiest pants known to mankind, and the next, pleather makes a surprising comeback from the 1970's. As a teenager you should be experimenting with your look and figuring out things you love. It's a time to dream big and think about what you want to do with your life.

But what if you never got to do that? What if, for one reason or another, your window of opportunity to be a "normal" teenager floated by and you were thrust into adulthood early on? That part of the human development process goes missing and you're left wondering what your life would have looked like if you had been given the opportunity to be a teen. You feel jealous of the people who did. You wish you had gone to prom and eaten crappy food. You wish that someone would have asked you to homecoming, or at least you could have stood in a gymnasium full over overdressed teenagers and latex balloons. Having the chance to be a Middle soothes all of these feelings and missed opportunities. You can wear the school uniform to see what it feels like. You can feel younger, vibrant, and free. You can play and experiment with a look that you've always been curious about during high school, but you never got to try. Under the care of your Dom/Domme, now you have someone who supports you in going into "Middle Space" to become that part of you that never got the chance to shine before.

Being a submissive, and being a Little is something that stays with you forever. It's a part of who you are and who you always will be. Just as your Dom/Domme will age and change, so too, will you grow, change, and age. Can you be a Little and be older? Absolutely you can! There will come a day when I will be rocking the gray hair and still I'll be singing every Disney song and wearing the cutest kawaii pajamas. But let's get real here for a moment. As the brain ages, your tastes within DDLG might change a bit and that's perfectly fine. Maybe wearing diapers at 65 is hitting just a bit too close to home, so you need to do something different for little space. This is where being a Middle would be an excellent fit for older littles.

Who doesn't want to feel younger, vibrant, hopeful, and optimistic? I know I do! Becoming a Middle allows you the freedom to be happy, surround yourself with cute things, while still being able to walk and talk with your caregiver. Like other groups within DDLG, being a Middle can also help aid mental health. You can look adorable and nerdy while rocking a fabulous cosplay outfit. The possibilities are endless!

What I don't want you to think is that Middles are like the fantasies depicted on porn sites. This simply isn't true, and as stated in the introduction, sex in little space is a choice between the dominant and submissive. Choosing to become a Middle simply means that you wish to regress to an age of adolescence. It's a mental shift akin to the movies, *"A Cinderella Story"* and *"13 Going On 30"*, where you can be young, wild, and free! You are sexy! You are adorable! You are desired! And you've *still* got it! Like the other branches within the DDLG community, becoming a Middle doesn't have to break the bank. So, let's take a look at some items that might enhance your play within Middle Space:

15 Tools to Help New Adult Middles on Amazon:

1. Littleforbig Cosplay Magic Onesie School Skirt Set- $39.99 USD
2. Sock It To Me Knee High Socks- $12.00 USD
3. Kawaii Polka Dot Backpack- $19.99 USD
4. Mermaid Tail Blanket- $21.99 USD
5. 12 Bath Bomb Set- $19.99 USD
6. Cat Paw Mini Skirt with Suspenders- $20.99 USD
7. Silicone Cat Night Light- $13.99
8. San-X Stationary Set- $19.99 USD
9. Unicorn Cosplay Onesie Pajamas- $23.99 USD
10. Tumbleweed Mug Set of 2, "I love you, I love you more"- $29.95 USD
11. Knaughty Knickers "It's All Yours Daddy" Panties- $13.99 USD
12. Znart 5 pack Cartoon Animal Socks- $11.99 USD
13. Heart Sunglasses- $9.99 USD
14. Miyang Indoor Slippers Fleece Plush- $19.99 USD
15. Gent House Love Lambs Sleep Mask- $11.98 USD

Quick Tips & Tricks To Care For An Adult Middle:
- Remember that your Middle wants to be able to verbalize their feelings even though they have regressed to a younger age. Allow them to be playful and express themselves.
- Take your Middle on many different trips to spark their sense of wonder and curiosity. This can range from sporting games to museums to free outdoor concerts during the summer. Go wild with it!
- Take your Middle shopping! It's likely that your Middle loves to get new things so a shopping trip to pick out new outfits and accessories for Middle Space is a great bonding activity. (Bonus points if you pick out the items for him/her to wear as you purchase items).

- Your Middle might be all about technology. Try giving your Middle a kawaii phone case as a surprise gift. These are available at many stores such as: Claire's and Justice. You can also pick out a personalized ringtone that is sure to make your Middle smile each and every time you call!
- Encourage your Middle to design their bedroom in a way that expresses their "inner Middle". Help them to pick out fun bedding, posters, etc. to create a little space that evokes happy feelings as they rest.

Things to Do to Make Your Middle Smile:

1. Have a video game night. There are plenty of MMORPG platforms and Co-Op games for you and your Middle to enjoy together. (I recommend getting a Steam account).

2. Have a Salon Date. Give your Middle the best pampering by scheduling a couple's salon date. You can even get fancy and get a couple's massage!

3. Make a scrapbook together. Nothing makes a little smile more than an arts & crafts project that you two can do together to capture all of the wonderful memories you've made.

4. Make tie-dye shirts together. With two cotton t-shirts, rubber bands, a bucket, and dye, you can let your little one gets super creative while creating shirts for you both!

5. Try new foods together. This doesn't need to be fancy or expensive. In fact, my Daddy and I love to go into our local grocery store and pick out frozen pre-made dishes that we've never tried and do a mini-buffet as a date night!

6. Take a Road Trip Together. This can be touring your local community and treating it as if you were a tourist, or you can mark places up and down your state and hit the road!

7. Go camping. What a cheap, but fun activity! Your Middle is sure to love sleeping beneath the stars, fishing, and cooking around the campfire with you. (There are some very cheap tent sites at RV parks so check them out online!).

8. Start a piggy bank and allowance. Teaching your Middle to save their money is also an important task to learn. Giving them a piggy bank and a small allowance is a great way to put them in the little mindset, while teaching them the value of saving a dollar.

9. Go see a favorite band in concert. Maybe scoop up a band t-shirt or two too!

10. Go to a drive-in movie. Snuggling together in the car while watching a movie is the best, and you can bake your own snacks to bring along to the movie too. It's a fun, cheap date to share all while catching the latest movies.

Chapter VI.

Budget Babes: The Top 50 Recommended Little Products Under $20 USD

*W*hen I was young, my parents told me that I had to get creative when it came to Halloween costumes. My mom would help and make my costumes at home when I was very young. But as I got older, they encouraged me to turn a simple cardboard box into various things: a time machine, a robot, or a toaster. One year when I was in our neighborhood 4th of July parade I dressed myself up as Benjamin Franklin, complete with gluing cotton balls to a shower cap to make a wig. Having to create things "on a dime" has long been a passion of mine. I'm a creative soul, and I know you can be too. One of the biggest mistakes that people new to the D/s scene make is thinking that they need to purchase many products up front to create a little space. This couldn't be farther from the truth.

I like to think of little space like an actor thinks of putting on a performance. You need to get into character. You set the stage and suspend your mind to slip into a different state of being. Improvisational actors barely use any props, yet their performance can easily captivate an audience because they infuse such passion into their actions and performance. The story comes alive and you feel gripped in the moment by their words and the sounds they make. So, too, can this translate into making a little space for yourself.

If you are blessed with tons of money, then honey, go to town and shop to your heart's delight! There are bunches of DDLG/LB products online to keep you stock for years to come. But if you're like me, and you need to make that penny stretch, well you've come to the right place. I love figuring out tips and tricks to circumvent having to buy many new things to get into little space, and now I'm happy to share them with you too. Let's take a look together at the five main categories of products that I think will help enhance your little space all without breaking the bank:

I. Health and Beauty:

Face Wash: Honey, nobody wants to kiss a nasty, greasy face whether you're in little space or not. But you don't need to buy a million face masks or slap 10 layers of goo on your face to keep your skin shiny and clear. Ditch the 10-step Korean skincare plan and instead head over to your local Target. For $3.99 USD, I use the Target Generic bottle, "Up & Up: Invigorating Facial Cleanser, Oil Free" that is the comparable generic brand to Clean & Clear Morning Burst Cleanser. It works fabulously and has those tiny scrubbing beads to exfoliate your pores. You'll be dancing in the shower the next time you scrub yourself with that cleanser.

Baby Wipes: I'll tell you a secret: when it comes to things going on around your private parts, do not skimp out and buy the cheapest of the cheap! Sure, you can go down to the dollar store and buy that half-dried up pack of baby wipes, but should you? Gosh no! We're talking about the most sensitive part of your body! No, you need to head to your local Walmart or Target, or you can even go online to Amazon and stock up on some Huggies Baby Wipes. For $10 USD you can get 500 wipes in bulk and your body will feel soft, clean, and refreshed every time you wipe. In the South we use them all the time since we're sweating up a storm. Trust me on this one, they're awesome.

Chapstick: My fellow female Littles, listen up for a moment. Men don't like having lipstick all over them when they kiss you. Lip gloss is far more tolerable to bear, but many men prefer a more natural look to their little. A bit of "natural looking" makeup goes a long, long way and Chapstick can do just the trick. I recommend Burt's Bees Chapstick, but there are many inexpensive brands on the market that will suffice. Slap on a little and pucker up for your Dom/Domme.

Kids' Toothbrush/Toothpaste: This is an easy, inexpensive area where you can feel little while still doing an everyday task like brushing your teeth. Children's toothbrushes often have soft bristles, which are beneficial for your teeth anyway. Pick out (or order online) a bamboo toothbrush and find a toothpaste that tastes good that you enjoy. Seeing it daily will remind you of being little and is sure to put a smile on your face.

Coconut Oil: I cannot tell you how much coconut oil has helped me in my everyday life. I cook with it. I rub it on my skin for lotion. I have used it on rashes since I have very sensitive skin. I use it in a DIY deodorant recipe. I could go on and on. For $18 USD you can purchase a pound of organic coconut oil at your local Costco Warehouse and be set for months. It's very much worth the buy because you can make many natural health and beauty products using coconut oil as a base.

Baby Powder: My Daddy loves the smell of baby powder, but beyond that baby powder is excellent for keeping your skin dry and soft. It's especially nice to have on hand for adult babies who do a daily diapering routine. Have you ever stepped out of the shower, dried yourself off, and then dabbed a bit of lavender-scented baby powder over your body and between your thighs? Yeah... the next time you try this I know you'll be hooked too!

Lavender Oil or An Essential Oils Kit: This is excellent to have on hand for many reasons. I recommend purchasing an essential oil kit off of Amazon for about $20 USD because the various scented oils can come in handy for different ailments. If you're congested use eucalyptus or tea tree oil. If you have an insect bite, tea tree oil or mint is very helpful. Tea tree oil also comes in handy to reduce inflammation in foot soaks. Lavender oil is excellent to soothe before bedtime and reduce stress. The power of gentle smells does wonders to set your mind at ease and help you to get ready to slip into little space.

Bath Bombs: Now you can go all DIY and make your own bath bombs, and yes, I have looked at the crafting videos too. But honestly, for $10 USD you can head over to Target and pick up a bag of mini-bath bombs already made and scented. I choose the later. If you've never taken a bath with one I encourage you to do so. Not only does your bath become colorful and fun, (the perfect little play space!), but it smells fantastic and makes your water relaxing to soak in.

A By The Tub Chair or Stool: This one can be completely free if you have a small step-stool sitting around your house. Instead of having your Dom/Domme crouch down on their knees to wash you, have them sit on a small chair or stool. This will make them comfortable as they wash you up, and it ensures everyone is relaxed during bath time. I can't slip into little space when I know my Daddy isn't comfortable. With a simple chair on hand and him comfortable, I can let my mind go and then have fun in the tub!

No Tears Water Pitcher: When I was compiling this list for you, I chuckled when I wrote this item down. When I was young I remember my parents telling me to just slap a hand over my eyes, or they would hand me a washcloth to cover my eyes right before they dumped a cup of water over my head in the bath. They would say, "Don't cry!" and then proceeded to wash soap all down my face and body. Nowadays they have pitchers for $10 USD that actually can be placed up against the forehead so that when you pour the water it goes back into the hair and not down into the eyes. It's much more relaxing and can be a great tool to use during little space bath time. Or you can grab a cup from the cupboard and do it "old school style". You choose, no judgment here!

DIY Deodorant
(Yes, this deodorant really works even when you're sweaty and extra funky!)

Ingredients:
2 tablespoons baking soda
1 (12 ounce) Mason Jar with a lid
1 jar of coconut oil

Instructions:
1. Place 2 tablespoons of baking soda in the jar.
2. Fill the rest of the jar with tablespoons of coconut oil until you reach near the top. Leave yourself about an inch of room to mix everything around in the mason jar.
3. Mix together until the baking soda is well incorporated. The baking soda will be the natural deodorizer and will remove any body odor you may have. The coconut oil will moisturize your skin. Use a small amount on your underarms as needed. Enjoy!

II. Toys:

A Baby Rattle: When it comes to buying toys for your little space, a baby rattle is an excellent place to start. Like a maraca, a rattle makes that rattling noise that draws your attention. As you shake it, you can't help but smile. It's as though the brain and body tap into a long-lost place of infancy where it distantly remembers shaking a rattle as a baby. You can easily slip into little space with the simple shake of a rattle, and for a few dollars you can purchase many cute rattles off of Amazon.

A Plushie/Stuffie: Everyone has their favorite stuffed animal or two. I sleep with my plushie dog, Mutsy and an elephant "Ellie" that I purchased at Kohl's. (Side note: Kohl's has a "Kohl's Cares" program where you can purchase a plush animal and 100% of the proceeds goes to help kids in need. Their plushies are so soft and well-made and it feels good to be giving back. I highly recommend them!). Go online or go out shopping at your favorite store and find a plushie that just draws you to it. You'll know when you see it, but it doesn't need to be something expensive. All you need is a plushie that you know you can snuggle to at night that makes you smile. Then you're set!

Binky/Pacifier: There are few things that will make you feel like a baby quite like a pacifier, but it can be tricky to find an adult pacifier at your local stores. I recommend heading online to Amazon and spending $8-10 USD to purchase a simple, adult DDLG pacifier. I chose to go with a pink pacifier by the company, LittleForBig, for $7.92 USD on Amazon. Their product is excellent and the binky has held up well over many months. The best part? It's plain plastic, so you can always put stickers on it, or bling it up with beads and a hot glue gun once it arrives! Make it your own!

Books: This is one area where you don't need to spend a penny. Head to your local library and stock up on a bunch of picture books! You can even make it a weekly ritual with you and your Dom/Domme and then have weekend story-time and snuggles. Doesn't that sound nice? :)

Chalk: Chalk is so much fun to play with, isn't it?! You can get out in the sun and create elaborate pictures from your wildest imagination as you draw for hours. Or, you can make a giant four-square and get a game going with your Daddy/Mommy. Or, you can play tic-tac-toe! When you're all done, pour some water on the ground and wash the slate clean. Then you're all set for more fun, artistic adventures!

Used Building Blocks: I say used here, because have you seen the prices on brand new building blocks? Honey, they are ridiculously expensive! No, this is one time to head to your local thrift shop, charity shop, or Goodwill and poke around in the toy section. All the time parents are donating used Legos, building blocks, etc. that you can purchase for a couple of dollars. Save yourself a bundle and go used with this item to have a toy on hand that is so much fun to play with in your little space.

Toy Cars: Toy cars are also a blast to play with! They are a great toy to have on hand in little space when you want to play but to keep things quiet in the environment. The tactile motion of rolling the car back and forth can keep a little occupied easily while your Daddy or Mommy is doing something else. Also, many toy cars have doors that open and shut which can allow for deeper creative play. While you can purchase a new toy car online or in the store for less than $20 USD, I recommend trying to find a used toy car in a charity shop first. Buy used, and save the difference!

Bouncy Ball: I remember when grocery stores used to have these large end caps with elastic bands all around the sides. From floor to ceiling there were colorful, bouncy balls inside. I remember looking at all of these balls longing to purchase one for a few dollars. Every once in a blue moon I got lucky and my parents picked one up for me. Oh, how much fun you can have with a bouncy ball! You can play kickball with your Dom/Domme. You can toss it back and forth or play an impromptu game of basketball. You can toss it up in the air and play catch, or knock it around like volleyball! For a couple of dollars, it's definitely worth the buy for many hours of fun feeling little.

Jump Rope: Jump rope is a great toy to have on hand to play with your caregiver. There is a company called, Amble, on Amazon that sells segmented, 7.5-foot jump ropes in various colors for $10.99 USD. I highly recommend this brand. In addition, there are longer jump ropes you can buy if you want to gather your little friends together for a game of "double dutch"!

Wooden Peg Dolls: Head on over to your local craft store and for less than $5 USD you can purchase a couple of wooden peg dolls. These plain, wooden dolls are wonderful for an arts project with your daddy or mommy. Make the doll how you want it to look. You make one of you, and one of your dom/domme! Think of how much fun it would be to play with your wooden peg dolls of you and your dominant inside a dollhouse? I know it would be a blast!

<u>**Quick Tips For Purchasing Toys For Little Space:**</u>
- Try buying gently used toys before you purchase new ones. The environment and your wallet will thank you.
- Search your local Craigslist to see if there are any toys you can get for cheap.
- Next, check your local charity/ thrift/ up shop to see if there are any toys that spark your interest.
- Lastly, get out in nature and think of natural, DIY toys that you can make! Sticks can become magical wands. River rocks can be painted to make pretty home décor for your little space. Old, corn husks can be dried and woven to become dollies. Sticks and rubber bands can make a slingshot! There are many crafts you can make gifts from nature. Just take the time to get out and explore your own backyard!

III. Essentials & Mealtime Products:

Bib: There are many adult bibs out on the market that cater to the elderly population, but few that are designed for the DDLG community. In my opinion, if you want to put a bib on your little for mealtime, simply tuck a napkin in around their neck. By doing the action for them, you're automatically setting the mood for little space and you don't need to spend any money to make it happen!

Sippy Cup: My biggest gripe about sippy cups before I found what works for me, is that either the straw was made to remain inside the lid therefore making me squeamish about getting it properly cleaned after use, or that the cup was made with a spout with small holes and it took forever to drink. My solution was to find a cup with a removable straw which I found at my local dollar store. Head to your local store and pick out a very, cheap sippy that costs next to nothing and save your money for bigger items (like apparel) to enhance your little space. This is one area where you don't need to spend much at all!

Plastic Kids Plate: You can find many excellent kids plates to use for mealtimes at your local dollar store, or any discount thrift store. People are ditching children's dinnerware all the time and this enables you to pick it up on a dime! Check out if there are any porcelain mugs with cute animals, or plastic princess plates, etc. You'd be surprised what people are tossing away. Remember: one man's trash is another man's treasure.

Finger Foods: This is probably the single most important thing to have on hand for little space during mealtime. Kids love to eat with their hands! As adults we naturally gravitate towards using utensils, but try incorporating more finger foods into your meals to create a meaningful, fun little space with your Dom/Domme. I recommend purchasing: chicken nuggets (regular or vegan), french fries, broccoli florets and cheese dip, goldfish crackers, Cheerios, bite-sized crackers, cheese cubes, vegan sausage links (then cut up into pieces), grapes, bananas (to mash or cut up), etc.

Placemat: I can't tell you why placemats are so expensive. I was recently looking online for some seasonal, autumnal placemats for my home. They wanted almost $40 USD for a set of four! My mouth dropped and I scowled in protest. Placemats for little space can easily be acquired for dirt-cheap at your local dollar store. Let the big brand companies keep their fancy placemats. You head to the Dollar Tree and save yourself a bundle of money!

DIY High Chair For Adult Babies: ABDL high chairs can easily run you into several *hundreds* of dollars, and honey this kitten doesn't have a money tree in the backyard! So, I came up with a creative solution for you to make your own ABDL highchair for less than $50 USD. Go online and purchase a "bedside eating table". On Amazon US, there is one by the company, Coavas, for $37.75 USD. It's a simple table on wheels that you can roll right up to a bed... or a chair! It's also adjustable so you can make the table work with your own chair! No need to buy an extra chair for this project. Next, grab your stickers and paints and go to town coloring and designing the cutest, most glittery table the world has ever seen. Tada! You now have your own personalized ABDL highchair!

Picnic Blanket: Going on a picnic is one of the easiest, and cheapest activities you can do with your dom/domme to have a special date day out. If you're worried about your picnic food getting spoiled in the heat, try whipping up a few Vegan dishes that doesn't require a cooler! No meat, no dairy, no stress. You can have a tasty, healthy, fun picnic right next to a playground that will bond you both and put you right into little space in no time flat. So, grab a blanket from home, a flat sheet, or any type of blanket you have on hand and get moving! (See the end of this chapter for five, excellent Vegan recipes to make on your next picnic!).

Mason Jar Nipple: As I explained in the previous chapter, bottle-feeding is an amazing activity to do with your caregiver. You can relax, and suckle your favorite drink all while being snuggled up and held by your dominant. There are few things more moving that will put you into little space like bottle-feeding. I have found that the best nipple for littles is a mason jar compatible nipple that is specifically (6 months +/ fast-flow). This allows milk to flow fast enough for you to take a mouthful every few seconds

Baby Utensils: For just a couple of dollars you can pick these up at your local Target or Walmart or even your dollar store. Baby utensils are fun to use and make feeding your little safe because the tips are usually rounded to prevent poking or hurting gums and teeth. So, if you're a daddy or mommy and you're new to feeding someone food, a set of baby utensils is a great, cheap tool to have on hand to enhance your little play space.

Snack Cup Carrier: These cheap cups can be picked up in your local dollar store. They are handy to have if you like having snacks with you as you're on the go or want to go for a picnic. The snack carrier lid is usually made of silicone and has a central opening to allow for you to reach in and pull out a snack without the snacks falling out while not in use. I highly recommend it for any active little!

Five Easy Vegan Recipes To Make For Your Next Picnic:

Rainbow Fruit Kebabs

Ingredients:

- Red fruit = chopped watermelon
- Orange fruit= 1 chopped orange
- Yellow fruit = 1 cup of chopped pineapple
- Green fruit = 1 cup of green grapes
- Blue fruit = 1 cup of purple grapes

Instructions:

1. Using large BBQ skewers, place the chopped fruit on each kebab in the order of the rainbow. Set into a Tupperware to pack into your picnic bag, and you're set! Enjoy!

PB & J Sushi Rolls

Ingredients:

- 8 slices of whole-wheat bread
- 1 cup of creamy peanut butter
- ½ cup of your favorite jam

Instructions:

1. Begin by laying out all of the pieces of sandwich bread.
2. Place peanut butter on 4 of the slices, and jam on the other 4 slices.
3. Combine into 4 sandwiches.
4. Trim the edges/crusts off of each sandwich with a knife. Then cut each sandwich into thirds to turn each sandwich into three long stripes.
5. Carefully roll each stripe up into a sushi roll and pack into a Tupperware for your picnic. Enjoy!

Chickpea Vegan Lettuce Wrap

Ingredients:

- 2 cans of chickpeas, drained
- 4 tablespoons Veganaise (vegan mayonnaise)
- 1 stalk of celery, washed and chopped
- a dash of paprika
- a dash of salt and black pepper
- 2 cups of lettuce, chopped
- 4 large burrito tortillas

Instructions:

1. In a mixing bowl, mash up the chickpeas finely to make a mush. (Using a food processor works wonders here, but if you're using a fork that's fine too!).
2. Add in the veganaise, spices, and celery and mix well. Then set aside.
3. Lay out the tortillas. Add a bit of lettuce and a couple spoons of chickpea mix. Then top with a bit more lettuce. Roll the wrap up like a burrito and seal it in cling wrap or aluminum foil. Set in a Tupperware to take on your picnic and you're set! Enjoy!

Vegan Pesto Pasta Salad with Cherry Tomatoes

Ingredients:

- 1 tub of vegan pesto (I prefer Trader Joe's Vegan Kale, Cashew, and Basil Pesto)
- 1 box of bowtie pasta or penne pasta
- 1 cup of cherry tomatoes

Instructions:

1. Cook the pasta according to the box. Then drain and set aside.
2. In a mixing bowl add the cooked pasta. Then pour in the vegan pesto. Mix well.
3. Slice the cherry tomatoes into halves and toss into the pasta. Mix well to combine.
4. Pour into a Tupperware and you're done! Enjoy!

Quick Tofu Pho in a Mason Jar

Ingredients:

- 2 (16-ounce) Mason Jars
- 1 pack mung bean/glass noodles
- 1 (32-ounce) carton chicken broth
- 1 tsp. Chinese Five Spice
- 1 tablespoon Sriracha
- 1 cup extra firm tofu, drained and cubed
- 2 tablespoons chopped fresh cilantro
- 1 tablespoon lime juice

Instructions:

1. In a pot warm your chicken broth. (Or vegetable broth if you're vegan or vegetarian). Add the Chinese Five Spice. Then add the Sriracha and lime juice. Bring to a gentle simmer then turn off the stove top.
2. In your mason jars, place the glass noodles at the bottom followed by the cubed tofu. (If you have any soft greens like spinach laying around you can add them here!).
3. Lastly, top the tofu with the chopped cilantro. Then pour the broth into each jar and seal with the mason jar lid. Now you have pho to go!

IV.: Apparel Items:

I want to mention a quick word about DDLG/LB clothing. As a plus size woman, it can be difficult finding clothing that flatters and makes me feel little, yet sexy. Believe me, I get it. As such, I designed this chapter into two parts: clothing you can wear out and discreetly be little, and clothing you can wear in little space being "out and proud". I also divided this chapter into a part for little girls and a part for little boys. I want *all* of the littles in our community to be represented. Lastly, you'll find some online clothing store recommendations where you can pick up these items that I suggest for your wardrobe. All of these stores carry plus sizes. If you happen to be thin, then God bless you and these stores are sure to have plenty of clothing for you to try. But if you have some curves or "fluff" (like me), then don't worry. I have the perfect set of stores for you to find clothing that is both colorful, cute, discreetly little, and fabulously stylish all while carrying our larger sizes! Enjoy this chapter and happy shopping, my friends!

Apparel For Little Girls:

- **Out & Proud Clothing Suggestions (i.e. Little Space Clothing):**
    1. Onesies
    2. Bloomers
    3. Knee high socks
    4. Skirts
    5. School girl uniforms

- **Discreet Little Clothing Suggestions:**
    1. Cardigans
    2. Uniform-esque dresses
    3. Bodysuits tucked under pants
    4. Character T-shirts (Hello Kitty, My Little Pony, etc.)
    5. Denim Overalls

- **Stores with Plus Sizes For Discreet Little Clothing For Girls:**
    1. Torrid
    2. ASOS
    3. Hot Topic
    4. SpreePicky
    5. RainbowShops

Apparel For Little Boys:

- **Out & Proud Clothing Suggestions (i.e. Little Space Clothing):**
  1. Onesies
  2. Character socks
  3. DDLB T-shirts
  4. Animal backpack
  5. Colorful athletic shorts

- **Discreet Little Clothing Suggestions:**
  1. Khakis
  2. Dinosaur T-shirts
  3. Fitted cargo shorts
  4. Skinny jeans
  5. Male choker

- **Stores with Plus Sizes for Discreet Little Clothing For Boys:**
  1. Hurley
  2. Littletude
  3. Kohl's
  4. Redbubble.com
  5. Target

V.: Media & Entertainment:

When it comes to media and entertainment, especially for Little space I am all about saving money. I refuse to spend money on cable TV normally. Why would I do it to watch little shows, right? Now I admit that I enjoy watching Netflix and there are plenty of children's programs and movies on there, so if you have a Netflix subscription then you have a vast selection of shows at your disposal. Below is a list of completely free, wholesome, positive, classic kids shows on YouTube for anyone to watch. I think they are all inspiring for little space because they each portray values such as: kindness, love, family, and friendship.

Here are my recommendations for the best, FREE little space TV shows on YouTube:

Oswald:
How can you not love this talking octopus, (voiced by Fred Savage), and his pet dog weenie... who is a hotdog! What I love most about this adorable show is that the background noise is gentle, classical music. It's soothing and inviting all while making you smile at this big, blue octopus with a tiny top hat.

Franklin:
This young turtle and his family go on many adventures together and is a show loved by many. This show is heartwarming to see Franklin's kind parents care for him and his sister as they hang out with their other woodland friends. I know you will love it too.

The World of Peter Rabbit & Friends:
This 1990's British show is a must-see for anyone who enjoyed the books by Beatrix Potter. Everyone knows that Peter was the naughty rabbit who went exploring in Mr. McGregor's garden. But did you know that there are many more adventures with Peter and all of the other creatures in the surrounding woods? Get swept away with this whimsical show as you sing the "Perfect Day" theme song.

The Wiggles:
This Australian show is a must-see for any little who loves to sing and dance. It's hard to not smile at all of the silly songs the Wiggles sing along with their friends, including an octopus and joke-cracking pirate! Before you know it, you'll be jumping up to dance along with each of their songs. Trust me.

Sesame Street:
Sesame Street is one of the most popular children's TV shows of all time. This American classic show is iconic to children across the globe. Sesame Street comes in many languages and teaches core values that anyone can appreciate. Relax in little space as you listen to Big Bird, Elmo, Grover, Bert & Ernie, Abby Cadabby, and many, many more!

Caillou:
This Canadian TV show is colorful and bright with a very catchy theme song. Caillou is a 4-year-old boy who loves adventuring and exploring. Sometimes he gets grumpy and his parents have to gently teach him how to work through his feelings, but at the end of the day, he is always ready to learn, love, laugh, and try again! I know you'll enjoy the primary-color animation as much as I do.

Peppa Pig:
This British TV show has a 24/7 live stream on YouTube for you to enjoy in little space. Peppa Pig is a young, female pig with a brother, mother, and father. She has many friends and loves to go to school. Any little is sure to laugh as Peppa snorts and figures her way out of problems and obstacles. The animation is beautifully drawn and it is still a very popular show on current TV.

The Berenstain Bears:
This 1990's cartoon American TV show has a catchy country jingle for every little to enjoy. This show follows the Berenstain Bear family as they navigate life in Bear Country living in a large tree house. Brother Bear and Sister Bear often get into mischief and try to find creative ways to solve their predicament! This show is sure to give you lots of giggles.

Arthur:
Based upon the books by author, Marc Brown, this American TV show follows elementary-aged aardvark, Arthur as he navigates his school and home life. Arthur has a bit more advanced topics (like going to the dentist, or going to visit the nation's Capital) to keep you interested.

Kipper The Dog:
This British cartoon show follows Kipper, a brown, curious, little puppy who loves to explore the world around him. It's a very soft, show with soothing sounds, perfect to watch just before bedtime.

Gullah Gullah Island:
This American 1990's live-action show follows a family on the fictitious island, Gullah Gullah, who love to laugh, dance, and hang out with their many friends. I loved seeing binyah binyah polliwog, their friend and island local, come over to play in his giant yellow frog suit. With all of the dancing and singing in his show, I know you will love it too.

Little Bear:
Little Bear is a wonderful show about a young bear cub who has many woodland friends. Reminiscent of Winnie the Pooh, this show also has soft sounds, and gentle sound effects to keep you tuned in without feeling overwhelmed. It's great to watch in little space while relaxing.

Chapter VII.

The Best Online and Print Resources for Littles

remember back when I first began my journey into DDLG. As a curious soul I wanted to research the lifestyle and learn more from other Littles. I wanted to read blogs, look at pictures, and watch YouTube videos. I wanted to understand what made littles be littles, and what kinds of daddies are out there. I wanted to know it all. But what I quickly discovered was that as much as there are DDLG websites out there that are informative and helpful, there are also many websites vilifying the DDLG community as well. There are people posting comments galore that spew hate and filth on an otherwise quiet, private lifestyle choice. It was all overwhelming and unnerving.

So, I made it my mission to help new littles not experience that same feeling that I had. In this chapter, I have compiled lists of authentic DDLG/LB blogs, tumblrs, Youtubers, and printed books for you to read. At the time of this writing (September, 2018), I have verified that each of these authors is still producing content for the DDLG/LB community. It is my sincere wish that you find these resources helpful and beneficial. I hope you make new little friends online (and who knows? Maybe you'll meet a dom/domme too!). And if nothing else, may you live and learn, laugh and love, and be your most authentic self!

- **DDLG Informational Websites & Forums:**
1. DDLG Forum: https://www.ddlgforum.com/
2. Littlespace Online: https://www.littlespaceonline.com/
3. The AB/ DL/ IC Support Community: https://www.adisc.org/forum/index.php
4. DDLG Friends: https://www.ddlgfriends.com/
5. FetLife: https://fetlife.com/
6. DDLG on Reddit: https://www.reddit.com/r/ddlg/wiki/resources

- **DDLG Blogs & Tumblr Pages:**
1. In Daddy's Arms: http://daddys-doll.blogspot.com/
2. DDLG Training: https://ddlgtraining.wordpress.com/
3. Living The Life In Love: http://livingthelifeinlove.tumblr.com/
4. Cumming Without Permission: https://www.domsub.life/
5. Sex With Emily: http://sexwithemily.com/
6. Lord Daddy 2: https://lorddaddy2.tumblr.com/
7. Daddy of the Den: https://daddyoftheden.tumblr.com/
8. Little Girl Lizzie: http://littlegirllizzie.tumblr.com/

- **DDLG Youtubers: (Check out their video content!)**
1. Havoc Rain

2. Stevop
3. Binkie Princess
4. The Little Princess
5. Alex Sparks
6. Little Moo Moo
7. Baby Bear Max
8. Princess Foxxie
9. Milkwebs
10. Edwin and Mina
11. Little Caia
12. Strawberry Milkies
13. Cutesy Unicorn Baby
14. Evie Lupine
15. Babydoll Peach
16. Littlesnookums
17. Lil Kitty's Littlespace
18. rileyslittlespace
19. Cotton Candy Princess
20. SweetFetish20
21. Back In Diapers
22. Littlelolikat
23. Toxic Kitten
24. Glitter Princess
25. Absolute Lunacy
26. Baby Cherry Pie (Spanish-speaking DDLG Channel)

- **DDLG Books To Have On Your Shelf:**
1. *"The Big Book For Littles: Tips & Tricks for Age Players and Their Partners"* By: Penny Barber and Mako Allen
2. *"The Age Play and Diaper Fetish Handbook"* By: Penny Barber
3. *"Diaper Discipline and Dominance"* By: Evelyn Hughs
4. *"There's Still a Baby In My Bed!: Learning to Live Happily with the Adult Baby in Your Relationship"* By: Rosalie Bent
5. *"Coffee With Rosie: Why Does My Partner Want to Wear Diapers?"* By: Rosalie Bent
6. *"Articles on Being an Adult Baby"* By: Michael Bent
7. *"The Adult Baby's Guidebook: The Life Struggles of the Perpetually Diapered"* By: Brian B.F. Burch
8. *"Adult Babies: Psychology and Practices: Discovering the structure, motivation, and needs of the adult baby"* By: Michael Bent
9. *"Littles: A Caregiver's Guide (BDSM Guides 101)"* By: Savannah Belle and Lyra Leigh

Chapter VIII.

100 Wholesome Dates for You and Your Caregiver
(Plus 47 Little-Inspired Recipes to Cook Together!)

I've always believed that the hearth is the center of the home. Long before I became a little, my Daddy (and husband) and I would love to cook together. We didn't have much money but we had a lot of love and big dreams. My wish for you, is that these 100 wholesome dates and 47 little-inspired recipes bring you and your Mommy or Daddy many moments of joy, laughter and love.

In the age of mukbang and being able to communicate over long distances easily, you can have dates for free or nearly free by utilizing technology creatively. You'll see that many of these dates will hardly cost you anything. I believe that the best dates come from working with whatever resources you have. If you have the means to go on a road trip with your caregiver, great! But if not, and you happen to be a solo little or your Daddy or Mommy is long distance, then never fear because I have the perfect list for you. Are you ready to get dirty, cook some delicious food, and have some great experiences? Then let's jump right in!

Date #1: Ice Cream or Froyo Date

If you've never been to a Froyo bar, you have to go! Seriously, is there anything more little than walking into a frozen yogurt shop clad in kawaii colors, picking up your little cup, filling it with that perfect swirl of ice cream. Then you and your Daddy or Mommy can choose all the toppings that you want! It's a fun, budget friendly, little excursion that I highly recommend.

Date #2: Bowling

Imagine laughing and squealing at your dom/domme as they wear those funky colorful bowling shoes, while you two share a slice of greasy yet delicious pizza. You can let your inner competitive side shine as you bowl frame after frame. Or you can head up to the arcade and test your hand at winning a new plushie. Bowling is an amazing little date activity to do together.

Date #3: Library Story Time

Most public libraries offer story time for toddlers and elementary age children. But that shouldn't stop you from making your own story time date with your Daddy or Mommy. In the quiet sanctuary of a library, you can curl up on a plushie chair, fill your lap with picture books and dive into an imaginary world. No one will look at you twice.

Date #4: Saturday Morning Brunch

There's something soothing and yet classy about brunch. First off, you get to sleep in which is always a win because you get extra snuggles with your Mommy or Daddy. But then you get to make breakfast mid-morning. And everyone knows that breakfast tastes amazing no matter what meal you are cooking it for. I recommend french toast!

Date #5: Fast-food Happy Meals

I'll let you in on a little secret as someone who worked in the fast food industry when I was a teenager: no one checks if you have a child in the car, if you order a happy meal. When you pull your car up through the drive thru line, they might ask you if you want a toy for a boy or a girl. Trust me, they're not going to check if you have a car seat in the car. So, not only will you save money by ordering a happy meal, but you get little sized portions too! Now I call that a win.

Date #6: Fishing Trip

Many people think that fishing is an expensive hobby to have. This couldn't be further from the truth. As a little, there is nothing more fun than squealing as you dig out a worm from the bait bucket, having your caregiver help you put it on the hook, and reeling in a fish. Be sure to check your local area to find out free places that you can fish or head to your local hardware store to get a cheap state fishing license. Many places will also allow you to rent fishing equipment. So, you can do this little date on a dime.

Date #7: Beach Day and Sand Castles

For the longest time, I didn't live near the beach and I always wanted to play on the sand and build sand castles. If you don't have access to a beach, I recommend having your dom/domme purchase a plastic kiddie pool, filling with inexpensive sand from the local store and you just brought the beach to you! Dance in that sprinkler, splash each other like crazy and make sure to take pictures. If you live near the beach, why are you reading this? Go! The ocean's calling!

Date #8: Camping Trip

There are a million things you can do with your dom/domme on a camping trip very inexpensively. You can cook over a fire, roast s'mores, go hiking, the list goes on and on. I think you'll find, that it is well worth spending $50 USD on a camp site to lay beneath the stars together.

Date #9: Slumber Party and Pillow Fort

Slumber parties are the perfect excuse to "Netflix and chill" while feeling little. In less than an hour, you can string fairy lights, grab a bunch of blankets and pillows, and create your own little nook to snuggle up together. While many would suggest watching a movie, I recommend taking this time to talk more intimately as dom-sub. You can put questions in a hat, or play "would you rather". With snacks and a sippy cup, this date is sure to be a hit!

Date #10: Coloring

Adult coloring books came about as a tool used for therapy and relaxation. So too can this activity be a calming date that you can do with your caregiver. There's something magical about zoning out while you color and the world is quiet. You know that your dom/domme is there coloring next you. And yet you're focused on creating this magical picture. It's a special date that you two can do together to make your world feel still and at peace.

Date #11: Bubble Bath with Toys

Bath toys are some of the least expensive items you can purchase as a little (see previous chapters for specific Amazon bath toy recommendations). I think it is a shame that American bathrooms generally don't have a tub big enough for two. So how do you get around this obstacle and create a date with it? You bring in toys. There are washable crayons for the bath that you and your dom/domme can use. You can use foam letters to play games together on the ledge and spell. There are ways to connect while one person is outside the tub and one person is inside the tub. This is your chance to take bath time to the next level!

Date #12: Feeding the Ducks

As I've gotten older, I realized that ducks are everywhere. Truly, everywhere. Go to the nearest lake in your local area and I guarantee there will be ducks (unless you live in Florida, in which case, they probably would have gotten eaten by alligators. Just kidding!). Feeding the ducks with your dom/domme is sure to bring a smile to your face and make you feel little while taking care of another living being. Go to your local dollar store to purchase several loaves of bread and you can easily do this activity for a half hour or more.

Date #13: A Trip to the Zoo

I both love and detest the zoo for many reasons, but ultimately had to include it in this list. The zoo can be expensive. However, it's also a swirling mass of parents with young children in chaos with ear shattering decibels. This is to your advantage, my fellow Little, because nobody is going to look at you as you skip down the path holding your dom/domme's hand (oohing and ahhing at every adorable animal). Is it worth it? I think so. It's definitely a date to put a checkmark next to on your little bucket list.

Date #14: Going to a Farm

I admit that I am partial to the farm. As a southern Little, I am going to try to win you over to do this date with your dom/domme. There are so many things to do on a farm. There are U-pick farms, farms with petting zoos, hay rides, baked goods, fresh ice cream and seasonal activities. You can wear your cutest overalls, get dirty, and still have a great time! And the best part? You can do this entire date under $20. I recommend http://www.pickyourown.org as a great site to find a farm near you.

Date #15: Drive-in Movie

Can we talk for a moment at how expensive the movie theaters have gotten? Not to sound incredibly old, especially since I am a Little, but $11 per ticket is slightly ridiculous. I love going to the movies just as the next Little, but for $11 I do not want to sit in a sticky, gum-filled seat that is uncomfortable and makes me feel like I'm being smothered by people. My solution: the drive-in theater! For several dollars less per person, you can see the current movies that are in the theater. But, here's the best part: you can bring your own food! No $5 colas or nasty popcorn for you, oh no. You can bring your little snacks (see recipes in this chapter) and eat amazing food, while watching your movie! How cool is that?!

Date #16: A Trip to the Mall

A big shout out to all my Middles for this date. You will fit right in with all the teenagers who love to go to the mall. As a Little, the mall can be a magical place. There is Build-A-Bear and the Disney Store. There are hotdogs on a stick and cookie shops in the middle of the walking area. There's even Dippin' Dots! The mall is a little's haven. It's air-conditioned, it's easy walking for all mobility, and your dom/domme is sure to not get bored. Go check it out.

Date #17: Farmers Market

If you've never purchased something in a farmer's market before, it can feel a bit overwhelming. But, you don't need to shy away from this opportunity for a great date because there are many things that take place in a farmer's market. There are free samples of food to try. Usually, there is live music from local bands and there are lots of artists and their works to peruse as you are walking around with your dom/domme. It's the perfect date to be Little and blend in to the vanilla world.

Date #18: Amusement Park

My Daddy loves roller coasters. I do not. If you're like me, where the thought of going 70mph upside down makes you want to scream and hide under a pile of plushies, never fear. Many amusement parks, cater to those who want to go on roller coasters and those who do not. Your dom/domme (or you) can get your adrenaline fix while you are tasting some amazing elephant ears. There are slower rides like a Ferris wheel and you're sure to laugh your head off in bumper cars. This is one date you do not want to miss.

Date #19: Water Park

Going to the water park or any body of water is the perfect excuse to show off your cutest Little swimsuit to your dom/domme. While most water parks won't let you slide down together, your dom/domme can easily be waiting at the bottom for you as you throw your arms up with glee, sliding all the way down to them. You can dance under a cascading waterfall or float on an inner tube down a lazy river. There are many fun activities to do together at a waterpark. Bring your sunscreen.

Date #20: Couple's Massage

You wouldn't think that a couple's massage as a DDLG/LB activity. This seems like something "Big Me" would want to do. However, laying side by side as a professional rubs the knots in your muscles away is the perfect date to relax you enough to go into little space afterwards. Trust me, you're going to like this one.

Date #21: Little Shopping

Shopping for Little items doesn't need to be an expensive date. In fact, one of my favorite Little shopping excursions that my Daddy and I did was heading to the dollar store and stocking up on $20 worth of Little accessories. Get creative with your dom/domme and find a store that is comfortable for the both of you so that the trip is a pleasurable experience.

Date #22: Cooking Little Foods

I included 47 recipes in this chapter because I feel so passionately about D/s couples getting in the kitchen together. Outside of these recipes, there are many Little foods that you can make whether together or solo. You can make funfetti cupcakes. You can bake dino nuggets on a pan. Your cooking level does not really matter when the recipes are so simple to begin with. The result is a great time and being rewarded with tasty Little food.

Date #23: Baking Together

Baking can seem a bit more complicated. You need to measure things precisely. You need certain pans for certain recipes. And most of all, you need patience! This is something most Little's lack. However, with your dom/domme creating the batter or dough, you as the Little can have all the fun with cookie cutters and rolling pins and getting covered in flour, all while ending up making a tasty treat.

Date #24: Scrapbooking

I'm always envious of those people who scrapbook really well. You know who I am talking about. The ones with stickers and glittery pens and the perfect quote by every name. I am not one of those people, and you shouldn't feel stressed if you are not either. I love scrapbooking because it's the lazy Little's way of documenting your relationship with your dom/domme. You can tape pictures, movie stubs, coloring pictures. or love letters all on a page, slap a border around it and call it a day. Its laziness while being cute...I won't tell if you don't!

Date #25: Going Swimming

If you never checked out your local community pool, I encourage you to do so. You don't need to be a swanky Kardashian with an infinity pool to go swimming with your dom/domme. Many community pools are free if you can show proof of living in that area. Other apartment complexes provide pools for their residents. So why is swimming so great with your dom/domme? Size doesn't matter when you're in the water. You can finally do that piggy back ride that you've always dreamed of, or be picked up like Cinderella and weight doesn't matter. You can be kissed underwater, or do a handstand, play Marco Polo, or ride on your dom/domme's shoulders. Swimming is a must for every Little.

Date #26: Hot Tubs and Spa Retreat

There are many resorts that offer hourly services for their hot tubs. This can be a great DDLG/LB activity because the hot tubs are private. While your dom/domme is relaxing and unwinding in the heat of the tub, you are splashing in the bubbles and jets. You can usually bring your own snacks (think Goldfish, cheese cubes, juice boxes, etc.). So, for that time that you have use of the tub, you can make it the perfect Little spa retreat.

Date #27: Coupling / Matching Clothes

In South Korea, there is a fashion trend called "Coupling". This is when a boyfriend and girlfriend dress alike. One thrifty way to achieve this coupling date is to head to your local thrift store with your dom/domme and find clothes that match. Your Little side is sure to shine as you see your dom/domme dress like you!

Date #28: Trampolining

This date is the perfect excuse to wear your kawaii socks. Check your local trampoline park for a schedule of their adult public jump hours. Often, these are at reduced rates. You and your dom/domme can bounce of the walls (literally!) as you laugh and tumble together.

Date #29: Road Trip

This date is excellent for any budget bracket. If you can't afford to do a road trip out of state, why not treat your local community as if you were a tourist. You and your dom/domme can make an itinerary together, pack a bunch of delicious snacks, jam to your favorite tunes and off you go! Bonus points if you take a picture at every destination point.

Date #30: Picnic

Back in Chapter 6, I shared several recipes that are perfect for bringing on a picnic. A picnic is a wonderful, free activity that you and your dom/domme can do that can put you into Little space. Choosing a spot next to a playground is the perfect opportunity to combine a Little activity and a picnic together to make a great simple date.

Date #31: Movie Night at Home

Whether you pick up a movie from a local Redbox, or stream something online, movie night at home is a great Little date to do together. Netflix in particular offers many Little shows for all tastes. Spice things up by taking turns choosing what to watch so you learn what your dom/domme likes to watch too. You can pause whenever "nature calls", and your dom/domme can hold your hand as you take a trip to the loo.

Date #32: Disney Marathon and Sing-A-Long

It should be a requirement for every dom/domme to know every Disney movie. Why? Because odds are good that your Little likes to sing every song to every movie. If you really want to make your Little smile, take this opportunity to purchase a Disney CD to keep in the car so in between your marathon date, while doing a junk food run, you can bust out the Disney songs together in the car.

Date #33: Karaoke and Mocktail Making

We are Littles and therefore are not allowed to drink. Our dom/domme can drink, but we cannot. However, you can make such a fun date out of making a mocktail version of your dom/domme's alcoholic beverage. Have you ever tried a virgin margarita? It's a delicious strawberry smoothie. Or how about a Virgin Bellini? That's fresh squeezed peach juice on ice! You're sure to feel Little as your dom/domme is sipping a glass of rum while you're having some apple juice. Don't forget to maximize the YouTube window so you can bust out the karaoke songs while you are playing bartender.

Date #34: Cosplaying

Let your inner nerd shine as you become your favorite cosplay character together. Imagine your dom/domme as Naruto and you get to be Hinata, all shy, cute and adorable. Maybe, you want to be Sailor Moon and your dom is Tuxedo Mask? You can even have your dom be Cloud while you be Tifa! The possibilities are endless and you end up looking cute together. Check out a local cosplay convention near you.

Date #35: DIY Home Photo Booth

I'm not going to tell you to take naughty pictures, but let your imagination wander here. If you are an adult baby, think donning a onesie and posing cute for your dom/domme. If you are a Little, you put on the cutest outfit you got, bat those adorable eyes, and strike a pose. If you're a Middle, put on that uniform, sit on your dom/domme's lap, and snap a selfie. Getting silly in front of a camera is a great way to loosen up together. And if your dom says, to shed a few layers, well...

Date #36: Mini-Golf

This date is a great Little activity for many reasons. You can choose the color ball you want. Your dominant can teach you how to hit the ball into the hole. You get to whack the ball into a clown's mouth or a windmill. It's a fun activity that gets you moving, while being able to have private time on the putt putt course together.

Date #37: Arcade

There is literally an arcade game for every personality type. You and your dom/domme are sure to have a blast as you find the game which resonates with you. If you've never tried skee ball, extreme hoop shoot, whack-a-mole, or mad racer. You need to find your local arcade, my friend, and go. Many Chuck-E-Cheese's cater to adults using their arcades as well as children. You can easily slip into Little space while playing with your dom/domme in a place like that. Gather up your tickets, and see what prize you get.

Date #38: Circus

There are many circus groups that travel all over the world. While many people assume that circuses are places of animal cruelty, I urge you to go online and find a traveling circus near you. Nowadays, many circus groups focus on contortionists, trapeze artists, clowns, dance performers, and motorcycle acts while staying away from animal performances. You can get the childhood thrill of enjoying the circus all while being snuggled up to your dom/domme.

Date #39: Matching Henna Tattoos

Littles are notorious for disliking pain. Unlike our fellow masochist submissives, we usually draw the line at spanking. So, when it comes to a permanent tattoo, unless that's your thing, it's not going to happen. However, henna tattoos are the happy ground between a permanent tattoo and a temporary stick on one. You can find a henna artist through local festivals or farmers markets, and the henna tattoo usually lasts about a week before it washes away. Now you and your dom/domme can get a tattoo together without the pain.

Date #40: Tandem Biking

I like to call this activity: Couple's therapy on the cheap. Why? Because you have to work together to get to where you're going. As Littles we have to listen to our dom/domme, which makes this the perfect activity to do together. While you're pedaling upfront your dom/domme is telling you where to go and pedaling from behind. It's a great bonding date to do together. Check out local bike rental places online to find a tandem bike for you.

Date #41: Hiking

Being Little while out in public can get uncomfortable quickly if there are a lot of people around. Within the DDLG/LB community we try not to make vanilla people uncomfortable when we are out and about. Hiking is the perfect solution for being Little outside while having privacy too. Go out and explore trails near you with your dom/domme and marvel at Mother Nature. You can hold hands, share water bottles, pack a bag of snacks, and bring your Little world into the great outdoors.

Date #42: Horseback Riding

This date is an excellent activity to try something new. There are many guides who will assist you and your dominant's riding level and experience. If you happen to have a partner who is larger than the weight requirement, you can easily have your dominant guide the horse (and you) as you are sitting in the saddle. As they hold the reins and walk with the horse, you two can talk quietly in Little space as you squeal with delight with every shift and motion the horse makes.

Date #43: Hayride

This activity is perfect for any mobility level. If you've never been to a hayride during fall at a local farm, you have to give it a try at least once. Relax on some hay bales or wooden benches as a tractor pulls you around the farm and you take in the sites. Most hayrides are free although some cost a couple of dollars. Either way, it's a great seasonal activity to do together.

Date #44: Pumpkin Carving and Corn Maze

Remember that pickyourown.org website? You can pick your own pumpkin for Halloween. You and your dom/domme can easily make a date out of carving a jack-o-lantern together. Most farms offer a corn maze that you can purchase a ticket to enter too. I love going in a corn maze because you usually go at night, with nothing more than a flashlight and a map. Hold your dom/domme's hand as you navigate the spooky 7ft. tall corn maze together. Look for a farm near you.

Date #45: A Parade

Attending a local parade is a great place to discreetly go into Little space. Everyone is focused on the parade so you can quietly babble and snuggle up to your dom/domme while taking in the sights. There are parades for every holiday. So, you can experience this date over the 4th of July, Christmas, New

Year's Day, or Thanksgiving. If you don't have a parade near you, try tuning into the Macy's Thanksgiving Day parade online. It is one parade you, as a Little, are going to absolutely love!

Date #46: Theater Performance

Tickets to the theater can quickly get pricey. However, you can easily achieve this date on a budget by checking out your local community theater, or high school performance. Many schools open up their shows to the public, so for a few dollars you can take in a show and have this fun date together. Bonus points if the show is a children's show.

Date #47: Comedy Show

Laughter is the best medicine for having a relaxing date. My Daddy and I went to the Jo Koy, show to see his standup comedy. While a comedy show wouldn't be thought of as a DDLG/LB activity, your Big Me side can appreciate the humor while your little me side is just happy to be out with your dominant. Ask your Mommy or Daddy what show they would like to see and go laugh the night away. It's memories you'll hold dear forever.

Date #48: Mini-Vacation

A mini-vay is perfect when you just need to get out. A mini-vay or mini-vacation is an overnight trip to a destination approximately an hour or less away. I encourage you to get a map and see what cities lie around you that are an hour or less away. Plan an overnight trip with your dom/domme to shake up your normal routine and try something different. A single night in a hotel isn't very expensive, you can also savor little time by utilizing the hotel's pool, gym, and doing late night fast food runs.

Date #49: RVing

Rving is the best of both worlds. You're "glamping" (glamorous camping) with a hot shower and bathroom, but you get the inexpensive RV spot for cheaper spot while being outside. Now you can camp and sleep in the comfort of a bed at the same time. There are many companies online that you can connect with to rent an RV. Check out a local place near you.

Date #50: Painting

This date has many possibilities. You can attend a local class with your dominant and paint a picture together at a winery's "Sip and Paint" class. You can bring this activity home and buy blank mugs from the dollar store to paint together. You can also get creative and paint each other! You can even spice things up with body paint and use each other as a canvass.

Date #51: Pottery Design Class

I love this date because you can feel like you are in the movie, "Ghost", as you mold clay with your dom/domme. Many studios offer pottery design classes very inexpensively. Create a bowl or cup together then return two weeks later to see the fired, glazed, and finished result.

Date #52: White Water Rafting

Get adventurous together with this fun, but safe date activity. There are plenty of professional rafting companies who will assist you and your dom/domme as you navigate the river together. If you are in to roller coasters or a natural adrenaline junkie this date is right up your alley. As you're bouncing along the white-water rapids, you have to paddle together to keep the raft steady. You and your dom/domme are sure to have plenty of laughs together. Don't forget your helmet!

Date #53: Thrift Store Shopping

Shopping at the thrift store is an amazing place to find DDLG/LB items. Many thrift stores will bundle toys in storage bins for a flat rate of $5 to $10. You never quite know what you're going to get in the bin, but that's half the fun of purchasing it together. In addition, you can often find playmats, used playpens, baby blankets, and kawaii clothing if you take the time and really dig through the piles. What is one man's trash is another Little's treasure.

Date #54: Aquarium Date

Channel your inner mermaid as you and your dom/domme head off to the aquarium together. Many aquariums have special exhibits where you can interact in the touch tanks, as well as sea animals being fed up close and personal. You and your dom/domme can take pictures next to jellyfish, or giggle at an octopus that is trying to camouflage against the rocks. It's sure to be a date you'll never forget.

Date #55: Sailing

Anchor away at your local marina as you and your dom/domme go sailing together. There are fewer thing more relaxing than cresting over the waves with the wind on your face. Sailing requires you to work together as you raise, and lower the mainsail, and listen to the captain's commands. Check out your local yacht club to get involved in Sailing 101 courses inexpensively.

Date #56: Whale Watching

I have to recommend the Pacific Whale Foundation in Maui, Hawaii for this date. Not only do they specialize in conservation, but they help to further research on whales with every ticket you purchase from them. There are many whale watching charters you can connect with, to experience this once in a lifetime date experience. Trust me when I say that when you see a humpback whale swimming beneath your catamaran in clear blue waters, it will take your breath away.

Date #57: Video Gaming

My Daddy and I are giant nerds, so I have to gush to you about MMORPG's (Massively Multiplayer Online Role-Playing Game) and Co-op (Cooperative) games. If you are new to the video game scene, there are plenty of games that you and your dom/domme can get involved in that are free or nearly free. Steam is the largest digital platform to finding excellent Co-op games to play together. However, I would be remiss if I didn't recommend the subscription free MMO game Guild Wars 2 to play together.

Date #58: Dance Party

If you can afford professional couple's dance classes, and you have the schedule to make it happen, you probably don't need my help in creating your own DDLG/LB date. This date is for every Little out there that has a full schedule, limited funds, or a child. There are tons of free videos on YouTube that are dance tutorials for you and your dom/domme can learn together. Make your own dance party, and have a blast with it in the privacy of your own home. Who knows? You just might love the cha cha.

Date #59: Going Out to Eat

Eating out really isn't specifically a DDLG/LB activity. Now what happens if your dom/domme chooses what you eat and orders for you? All of a sudden, the mundane activity becomes a part of magical Little space. Not only do they order for you, but when the food arrives, they cut up your food for you before you begin eating. There are plenty of ways to enhance eating out as a Little activity. If you're really creative, look for a breakfast restaurant and see if you can order a smiley face pancake or something whimsical and playful.

Date #60: Candy Shop

Every Little has dreamed about Willy Wonka's Chocolate Factory. While the factory isn't real, we can experience the joy of being surrounded with sweet confections by visiting a candy shop. If you are a Harry Potter fan, you can choose various jelly beans to make your own Bertie Bott's mystery jelly beans, or you can get the thrill of licking a lollipop as large as your face. Your inner Little is bound to be elated at this simple yet fun date activity.

Date #61: Exercising

Many dom/dommes create rules for their Little that center around healthy living. Exercising as a D/s couple, makes you feel good because of the endorphin boost but it also is a great excuse to have a bubble bath afterwards. Exercising can range from something as simple as taking an evening walk together to trying couple's Yoga. Wear something comfortable and get moving!

Date #62: Role-Playing Online

If you've never roleplayed online before, it is akin to a choose your own adventure book. However, unlike the books, you weave the story. Just as an actor becomes a character on stage, a role-player becomes the character online. There are dozens of MMORPG's available with beautiful virtual worlds that you and your dom/domme can interact in with your characters. Design your character just like dress up, and let your imagination run wild as you enter the online universe. I recommend websites like "https://mmos.com/gamelist" as a guide to finding the right RPG for you.

Date #63: LARPing

LARPing stands for Live Action Roleplaying. There are many LARPing communities internationally that you can find information for online and get involved with. If you are creative and enjoy the thrill of becoming a character in a fantasy world,

this is an excellent date for you and your dom/domme. Events are usually held at camp grounds over the course of a weekend. Participants check in to the cabins on Fridays, eat dinner and then the game begins. As you wield your nerf sword and bean bags, you race across the campgrounds slaying down monsters while acting out your character. If you and your dom/domme are nerds, this date is a must try.

Date #64: Tea Party

A tea party is a Little's wonderland. You'll note in this chapter that there are several recipes perfect for a tea party, including scones, tarts, and buckeyes. A tea party doesn't have to be expensive or elaborate to look fancy and put together. There is something adorable and whimsical about putting mismatching patterns together and having various teacups at the table. Don't stress over having your tea party looking uniform and like that of a magazine picture. Instead, grab your plushies, a few cups and saucers, your favorite snack and your dom/domme and have a tea party.

Date #65: Christmas Tree Decorating

What Little doesn't like Christmas? You can get extraordinarily creative at decorating your tree for Christmas. You can make a DDLG/LB Christmas tree by hanging up pacifiers, baby bottles, and little rattles on the boughs of the tree. You can also buy an artificial tree that's pink or blue! As you snuggle by the fireplace, with your tree glowing in the room, it's sure to be a very special Christmas.

Date #66: Gingerbread House Decorating

Don't stress yourself over trying to bake, cut and shape a gingerbread house. Head to your local store during the holiday season and purchase a gingerbread decorating kit. You and your dom/domme can dream up the most magical house to design together with frosting and candy. Bonus points if you make it a DDLG/LB gingerbread house!

Date #67: Fashion Show

You've saved, scrimped, and collected all of those Little clothes in your closet. Your dom/domme loves to see you all dressed up in all Little clothing. Why not put on a fashion show for them? Strut your stuff using the hallway as your catwalk, twirling to music, and have fun with it. I have no doubt your dom/domme will smile.

Date #68: Card and Board Games

Board games are so inexpensive these days. There are many board games to tap into Little space including: Candyland, Jenga, High Ho Cherry-O, Chutes and Ladders Hungry Hungry hippo and Guess who. There are card games such as: Uno, Go-Fish, War, and Exploding Kittens that are inexpensive and can create a great date night in with you and your dom/domme.

Date #69: Go to a Car Show

If your dom/domme is into cars, this date is perfect for you. Have your dom/domme teach you a thing or two about cars, as you walk around this free event together. As a Little, you can marvel at old-fashioned model T's, roadsters, modified street racers and more.

Date #70: Attend a Christmas Light Tour

You can go on a paid Christmas light tour, or you can do it on the cheap like I do. Grab your dom/domme and a couple of thermoses of hot cocoa, then pile in the car. Drive around on Christmas eve and see which houses have decorated their house with lights. There's always a radio station playing Christmas music 24/7 to listen to. This free activity is so much fun to ring in Christmas together.

Date #71: Backyard Barbecue

If you don't have a fancy grill pit in your backyard, or you only have a small balcony instead of a backyard – you can still have your own barbecue. Nothing screams summer more than barbecued food. Imagine standing at the grill with your dom/domme right behind you as they hold your hand guiding the spatula to flip over the burgers. You roast corn together, mix the potato salad, and eat homemade popsicles. Whether you are grilling outside or in your tiny kitchen, as long as you are together, that's all that matters.

Date #72: Puppet Show

There are many centers for puppetry arts located all around the world. This lesser known art form is a wonderful venue for dominants and their Littles to attend. You don't need to be an actual child to appreciate the talent that puppeteers put into each performance. Littles will marvel as these puppets come to life singing and dancing to numbers. Don't have a puppetry art theater near you? Watch an episode of Sesame Street on YouTube, or make sock puppets together and put on a performance of your own.

Date #73: Botanical Gardens

You and your dom/domme can visit your local Botanical Garden to walk around and learn about different plants. Stroll hand in hand as you witness butterflies, bumblebees, and wild flowers galore. Most Botanical Gardens are free, or some might ask for a small donation. Check out one near you.

Date #74: Body Painting

I love a date that combines improving self-image with DDLG/LB. As a plus-sized Little, I feel that body painting allows you to get comfortable with your body while exploring your dominant's body. Ask your dom/domme to paint on you, while telling you all the things they love about your shape. Before you know it, you'll be falling in love all over again.

Date #75: Gardening

You can start a garden with your dom/domme by making a simple herb garden or a window sill flower box. If you have the room, you might want to try to create a small vegetable garden outside. Gardening has been proven to be a very relaxing form of exercise for people of all ages. Test your green thumb and see what you can grow today.

Date #76: Go Christmas Caroling

I admit, I am a bit of a Christmas junkie. Do you know the Christmas Carol "Here we come a Wassailing"? It's based upon Christmas carolers who would drink wassail to keep warm as they went from house to house. Many people are shut-ins for the holidays or unable to get outside for the holiday cheer. You and your dom/domme can make things a bit more magical by connecting with local organizations to go caroling. How much fun would it be to sing carols with your dom/domme in the snow!

Date #77: Making Pancake Art

Pancake mix is very inexpensive and this fun art form is a great date to do together. If you can find condiment bottles at your local dollar store, I highly recommend using them over Ziplock bags. Mix your pancake batter together, then add a few drops of food dye, place into the bottles and pour your design onto a hot griddle. Laugh together as you make hello kitty, Pokémon, Mickey Mouse, and more!

Date #78: Make a Snow (or Sand) Man

I don't have the luxury of snow where I live. I envy those that are able to build a snowman together. You and your dom/domme can gather sticks and old clothing. Don't forget the carrot! Then you can create and amazing snowman together during the winter months. However, if you live in a mild climate like I do, get out to the beach and build an epic sandman. Kelp can become the hair, driftwood can become the arms, and seashells can become the eyes. He can even have a mussel nose! It's not Frosty but it still can be a great date.

Date #79: Go Sledding

Many people think that you need to purchase an expensive sled to go sledding. However, you and your dom/domme can use many household objects as makeshift sleds. Sit between your dom/domme's legs on a trash can lid as you slide down the hill together. You can also use baking sheets or plastic inflatable inner tubes. They work wonderfully.

Date #80: Go Ice Skating

Every Little dreams of being a figure skater. Who wouldn't after watching Olympic skaters gliding and twirling around the rink? However, I like to think that this date is more like the movie "Serendipity", where you and your dom/domme are holding hands, waddling along the ice hoping not to fall down, as you laugh and cling to each other. This is one date you don't want to miss.

Date #81: Start a Collection Together

Collecting something with your dom/domme can be loads of fun. It could be anything like stamps, shells, toys or even drawings. The act of collecting will make you feel closer because you are both working towards a common goal. It's very satisfying to snuggle up and admire your collection as a culmination of both of your efforts.

Date #82: Create a Playlist

Back in the day, we recorded cassette tapes together. Then it was burning CD's together. Now, you and your dom/domme can create a digital playlist together. This date only takes an hour or so, but the playlist that you create is something you can enjoy again and again. Explore each other's musical taste and see what you discover.

Date #83: Breakfast in Bed

This date I something to pull out once in a great while. You don't want to be busting it out every weekend, or else it will cheapen the experience. Your dom/domme is sure to smile and shower you with tons of kisses when you surprise him/her with breakfast in bed complete with a loving note. Get creative with breakfast by using cookie cutters and shaping fruit into a smiley face.

Date #84: Snuggles & Siesta

Nap time is an important part of Little's weekend schedule. Weekends are the time when you can slow down and take a nap together. Become the little spoon to your dom/domme's big spoon as you rest, recuperate and rejuvenate together.

Date #85: Hibachi Grill Date

Hibachi grills are an amazing Little date because Hibachi chefs put on a performance with elements of excitement and intrigue. Marvel as the chef creates a flaming onion volcano, flips shrimp into his hat, juggles eggs, and does a whole circus routine with your food. Littles love playing with their food so this date is sure to be a hit.

Date #86: Build-a-Bear

Plushies are a Little's best friend and this store takes it to the next level. Create a plushie together and watch your Little kiss its heart as the assistant sews it up. You can even record your voice to put inside the plushie for your Little to cherish forever. I highly recommend this date as an activity to do together. If you don't have a Build-A-Bear near you, they have bears online to choose from and customize to your heart's content.

Date #87: Surfing and Paddle Boarding

This date is a great activity to do even if you are beginner surfer. Many surf schools will rent boards inexpensively by the hour for you and your Little to use. Learn to catch a gentle wave, and keep your balance as you take a lesson from a surf instructor. You can find a gentle beach or marina to paddle board side by side.

Date #88: Indoor Skydiving

Dominants are all about keeping their Littles safe and protected. So, jumping out of an airplane is probably not happening. However, if you want to feel like you're flying together, check out indoor skydiving. There are certified instructors to guide you in the wind tunnel as you learn to shift your weight while being suspended in the air. Think happy thoughts as you and your dom/domme become as light as a feather.

Date #89: Stargazing

This date is more than just looking at the stars. Connect with your local astronomy group or bring your own telescope as you discover: constellations, moving planets, shooting stars, meteors and more. Your Little will love finding the Big Dipper while snuggled up in your arms.

Date #90: Snorkeling

Witness marine life up close and personal in this relaxing undersea adventure date. Be Ariel for the day, as you hold your dom/domme's hand swimming around looking at fishies. See if you can find starfish and crabs. Snorkeling equipment is available for rent for less than $10. Check a surf shop near you.

Date #91: Food Truck Tasting

Many food trucks network together to create outdoor food courts. You can find most food trucks on social media. Make it a fun date as you taste a nibble from truck to truck, exploring as you go. This fun culinary date is sure to leave you smiling with your bellies nice and full.

Date #92: Have a Very Merry Unbirthday Party

364 days a year, it is an ordinary day. But one day a year, you get a birthday. Which means, you have 364 chances to have an Un-birthday party! Inspired by "Alice in Wonderland", you too can have a wacky tea party complete with an un-birthday cake all while singing the song! (Check out YouTube to hear the song).

Date #93: Attend a Sports Game

Attending a sports game is 50% about the team you are cheering for and 50% about the experience of being there. Yes, you and your dom/domme can wear matching jerseys while cheering for your team, but we all know that being in an arena is really where the fun's at. You have the kiss cam that makes every cheer, the stadium wave that gets you out of your seat, music that pumps you up, and endless flow of beer and greasy food for you to nosh on. Ask your dom/domme to take you out to the "old ball game".

Date #94: Read Bedtime Stories

A vital part of every DDLG/LB relationship is creating traditions and rituals together. One meaningful tradition that your dom/domme can do is establishing a bedtime routine with his/her Little. Reading a bedtime story calms the mind and directs their focus. It evokes imagination as you're slowly lulled to sleep and eases the body into peaceful slumbers to rest and repair for the new day. Create this important routine together by visiting your local library weekly to pick out picture books!

Date #95: Pet Store Browsing

Taking your Little to a pet store to ogle and enjoy little furry pets is sure to bring a smile to their face. Watch them squeal at the cute puppies and kittens and see their eyes widen as they point at the turtle trying its hardest to hide. Hold your little close as you look at birds of every color and snakes coiled up beneath a log. Watch them gasp at the furry bunnies and hamsters that scurry to and fro. Pet store browsing is a free activity that can mimic a wild safari experience.

Date #96: Bottle Feeding & Rocking

Bottle feeding while rocking your Little one, then burping them right afterwards allows dominants to establish a strong connection. The act of feeding and rocking allows the Little to feel safe and coddled helping them to regress deeply into Little space. It forms a very strong bond between the dominant and their Little because it is a gift of nourishment and love. It allows the Little to be vulnerable and open while giving the dom/domme the freedom to truly assume the caregiver's role.

Date #97: Kite Flying

You and your dom/domme can check out your local dollar store to purchase an inexpensive kite or there are many free plans and tutorials online. This windy day activity gives your Little a chance to feel as if they are in the movie "Mary Poppins". Many communities have kite flying festivals in the early Spring. So be sure to check online to see if there is one near you!

Date #98: Dancing in the Rain and Puddle Jumping

Some people think that the rain prevents you from going out to play. But every Little and their dom/domme knows that a rainstorm means its time for a whole new adventure! Grab your rubber boots and raincoats as you set off together jumping in puddles and dancing in the rain. Try to catch raindrops in your tongue or pretend that you are Totoro as you march along in the blustery day.

Date #99: Develop a Lovies Routine (Pampering Your Little)

Personal hygiene is paramount which is why many dom/dommes instill rules for their Littles to keep clean. Dominants can keep their Littles happy by getting involved in their hygiene routine. With a box of diaper wipes, some baby powder, and a towel, you have everything you need to keep your Little one clean and healthy. This activity allows your Little to feel comfortable getting more intimate with you as you touch their body in positive, gentle ways.

Date #100: Find the Perfect Plushie Together

A Plushie is a Little's best friend. As you tuck your Little in every night, you'll see them smile as you give a kiss to their plushie and a kiss to them. Just like adopting a pet, your Little will find a Plushie that speaks to them and connects with them in a deeper level. They say a Plushie chooses the Little and they choose for life. That is why, your dom/domme must treat your Plushie with as much love and respect as he/she does you. Finding the perfect Plushie is the best gift one can give a Little because you are giving him/her a best friend for life.

Tiny Treats:
47 Little-Inspired Recipes for You and Your Dominant

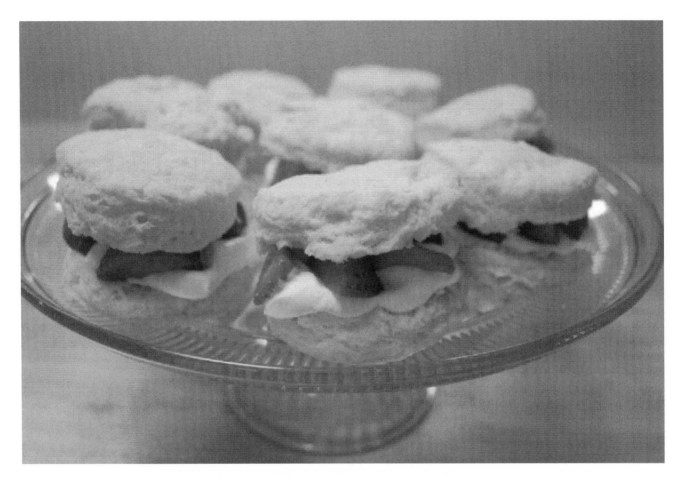

These scones are the perfect treat for any tea party. Pair them with a bit of whipped cream and berries and they taste simply perfect.

Penny Berry Scones

Serves: 16 scones

Ingredients:

For the Scones:

- 3 cups self-rising flour
- 2 cups heavy whipping cream/ thickening cream

For the Clotted Cream:

- 1 cup heavy cream/ thickening cream
- 1/3 cup sour cream

- 1 tablespoon confectioners' sugar

Additional:

- 1 (8 ounce) package strawberries, hulled and diced

Instructions:

For the Scones:

1. Begin by preheating the oven to 400 degrees F/ 200 degrees C. Combine the whipping cream and self-rising flour together. Form into a sticky dough.
2. On a floured surface roll the dough out to 1 1/2 inches thick then cut into rounds with a biscuit cutter or a drinking glass. Place scones into a baking sheet with a piece of wax paper.
3. Bake in the oven for 15 minutes. Then set aside to cool.

For the Clotted Cream:

1. In a stand mixer with a whisk attachment, pour in the heavy cream and whip until stiff peaks form.
2. Remove from the mixer and hand whisk in the sour cream and confectioners' sugar until just combined. Store in the fridge until you're ready to serve.

To Assemble:

1. Slice a scone in half. Place a tablespoon of clotted cream on the bottom of the scone. Add a bit of chopped strawberries on top of the cream. Place the top of the scone on and serve immediately. Enjoy!

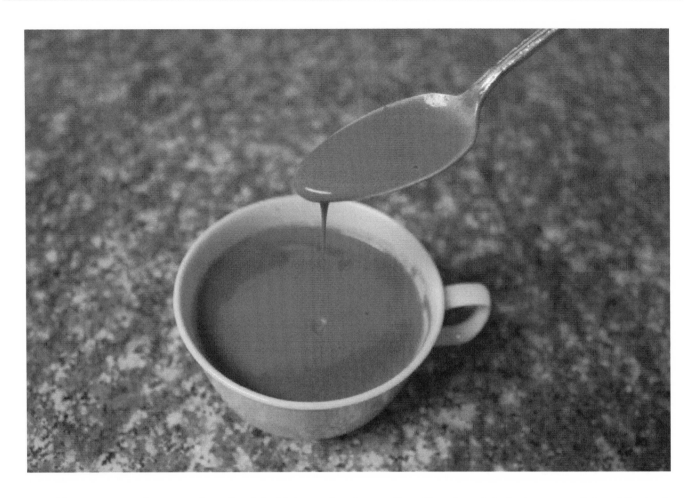

Hot cocoa can be exceptionally rich. This version keeps the silky chocolate taste you enjoy, while toning down on the sugar.

Kitten's Cocoa

Serves: 4 small cups or 2 larges

Ingredients:

- 2 cups of whole milk
- 5 ounces (130 grams) bittersweet chocolate, finely chopped
- 2 tablespoons brown sugar

Instructions:

1. Gather your ingredients.
2. Put a saucepan on medium heat. Meanwhile chop up the chocolate.

3. When the milk is warm, whisk in the chocolate and brown sugar. Continue to whisk for 2-3 minutes over medium heat. Be careful, it might froth up. If so, that's okay, just turn down the heat a little. (It will thicken up, just keep at it!).
4. Pour into tea cups and serve immediately. Enjoy!

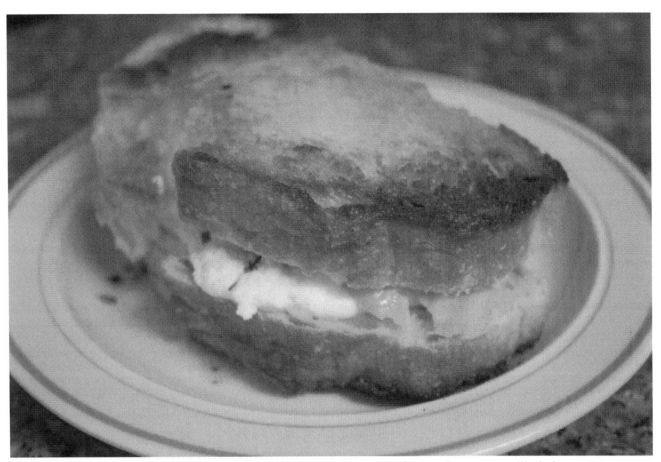

These sandwiches are sure to make you swoon the next time you're craving some grilled cheese. Be generous when buttering the bread to achieve that extra crisp.

Fancy Sammies

Serves: 4-6

Ingredients:

- 1 loaf of crusty, artisan French bread
- Butter
- 1 packet of chives, chopped
- 1 (8 ounce) tub of ricotta cheese
- 1 (6 ounce) package of smoked salmon

Instructions:

1. Gather your ingredients.
2. Place butter on the outside of each bread slice. (Go as generous as you want with it. No judgment here!) :). Then place in a hot skillet over medium-high heat.

3. While the bread is toasting use a spoon to put about 3-4 tablespoons of ricotta cheese and a sprinkle of chopped chives on both sides of the bread. Cook for about 2-3 minutes, or until crispy. Then lay a piece of smoked salmon on the right side of the sandwich. Use a spatula and spoon to carefully flip the top piece onto the bottom piece. Gently press together.
4. You can cut it in half and stick it in a brown bag for little hands like I did
5. Serve hot and enjoy!

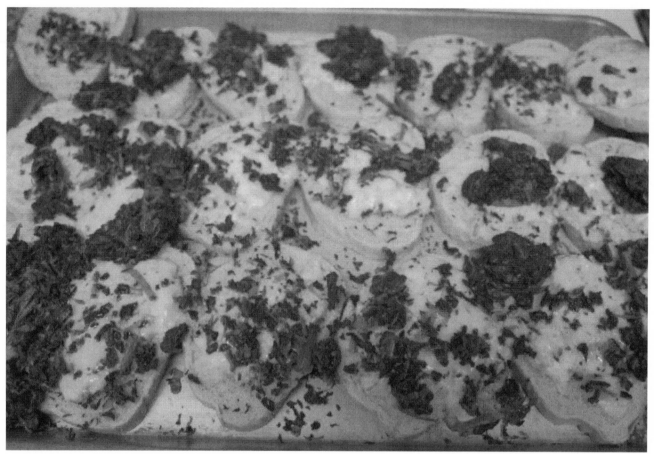

Get your greens in with this easy, cheesy appetizer. It's perfect for sharing with your Little friends.

Baby Baguette Bites

Serves: 6-8

Ingredients:

- 1 (8 ounce) bag of frozen spinach defrosted
- 4 tablespoons butter, softened
- 2 tablespoons minced garlic
- 3 cups shredded Mozzarella cheese
- 1 loaf baguette, sliced

Instructions:

1. Preheat the oven to 400 degrees F/ 200 degrees C/ Gas Mark 6.
2. In a small mixing bowl combine the butter and garlic and mix well. Then add the cheese and mix until it's a sticky paste.
3. (Now I used kitchen gloves for this part but feel free to get messy lol). Lay out a baking sheet and place slices of bread all over it. Then spread a bit of butter–garlic–cheese mix on each piece of bread.
4. Then press down some defrosted spinach into the mixture to make it stick together.
5. Bake for 10-12 minutes or until just golden brown on the edges.
6. Serve hot and enjoy!

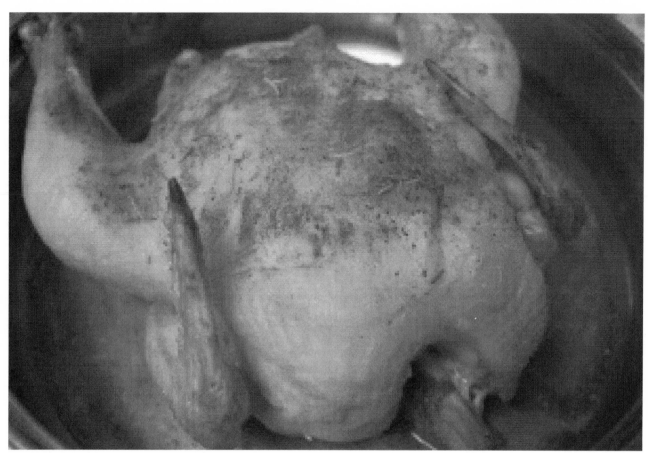

You can always catch me singing in the kitchen when I roast a whole chicken. To remember which herbs, you need just sing the Simon and Garfunkel song.

Scarborough Chicken

Serves: 1 whole chicken

Ingredients:

- 1 whole chicken, cleaned and rinsed
- 1 tbsp. dried parsley
- 1 tbsp. dried sage
- 1 tbsp. dried rosemary
- 1 tbsp. dried thyme
- 1 tbsp. Old Bay Seasoning
- A generous drizzle of olive oil
- Salt and pepper to taste

Instructions:

1. Preheat the oven to 425 degrees (F).
2. Clean, rinse, and pat dry your whole chicken. (If there are any innards, discard or save for frying up for another recipe).
3. Place the chicken in a deep saucepan. Drizzle with olive oil to coat the chicken. Then sprinkle on all of the dried herbs, Old Bay Seasoning, and salt and pepper.
4. Cook for 15 minutes on 425 degrees (F). Then when the timer dings, don't open the oven. Reduce your oven to 375 degrees (F) and continue cooking for 1 hour.
5. Let stand for 15 minutes to cool, then carve and enjoy! ☒

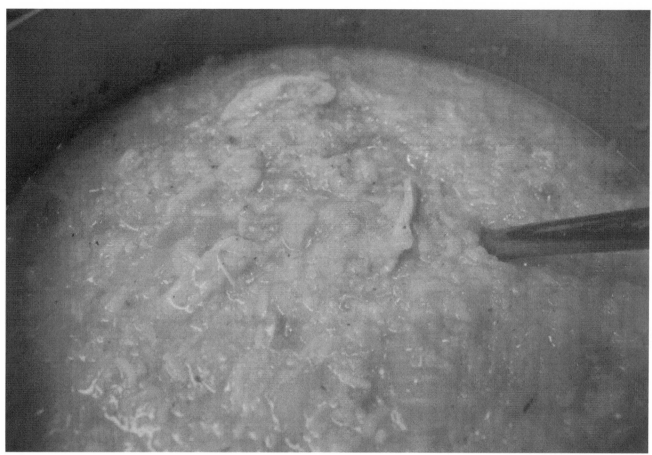

This bowl of rice porridge is perfect for when you're feeling under the weather or you've had a long day. Feed this to your Little for a fun play session food.

Cure-It-All Baby Porridge

Serves: 6 servings

Ingredients:

- 2 tablespoons olive oil
- 1 onion, diced
- 2 cloves garlic, crushed
- 1 (2-inch) piece ginger, peeled and thinly sliced
- 2.25 lbs. chicken wings, split and tops discarded
- 1 tablespoon fish sauce
- 6 cups chicken broth
- 1 cup glutinous sweet rice
- salt and pepper to taste
- 1 green onion, chopped
- 1 lemon sliced (optional)

Instructions:

1. Heat the olive oil in a large pot over medium heat; cook and stir the onion, garlic, and ginger in the hot oil until fragrant, about 5 minutes. Add the chicken wings; cook and stir together for 1 minute. Stir the fish sauce into the pot, cover, and cook another 2 minutes.
2. Pour the chicken broth into the pot. Add the sweet rice and stir. Bring the mixture to a boil; cover and cook for 10 minutes, stirring occasionally to assure the rice is not sticking to the bottom of the pot. Season with salt and pepper. Garnish with the green onion, and serve with lemon slices and additional fish sauce, if desired.

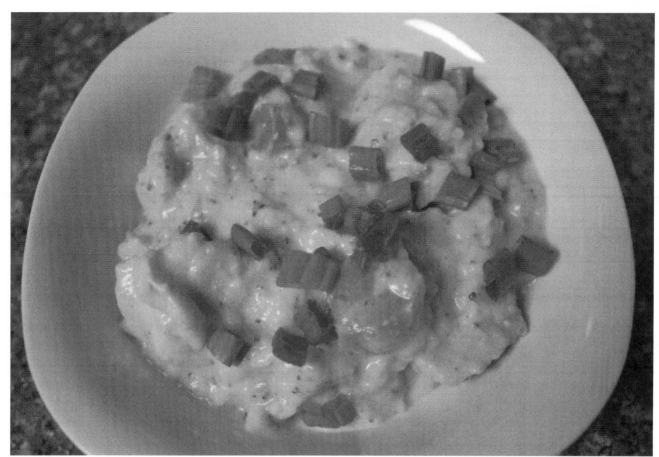

Hide your vegetables in this chicken stew that takes rice porridge to the next level. It's thick, creamy, and comforting. I know you'll enjoy it!

Chicken and Broccoli Chowder

Serves: 8

Ingredients:

- 4 boneless, skinless chicken breasts, cut into chunks
- 1 (16 ounce) bag of frozen broccoli florets
- 3 carrots chopped
- 1 onion, diced
- 8 cups water
- 1 pinch of dried sage
- 1 pinch of dried rosemary
- 1 pinch of dried thyme
- a few dashes of salt and black pepper to season
- 3 tablespoons chicken bouillon powder
- 4 tablespoons butter

- 4 tablespoons all-purpose flour + 1 tbsp. chicken bouillon
- 4 cups milk
- Leftover rice* (Optional)

Instructions:

1. In a deep soup pot place in the following: chopped, raw chicken, broccoli, carrot, onion, water, dried herbs, salt and pepper, and chicken bouillon. Bring to a boil, then reduce to a simmer. Cover the pot with a lid and cook for 1 hour.
2. After an hour, in a separate saucepan make a chicken gravy. Begin by melting the butter and then adding in the flour to make a roux. Then add in 1 tbsp of chicken bouillon powder and mix. Add in 2 cups of milk and continue to stir over medium heat until the gravy has thickened. Then add the additional milk and continue to stir until everything is a nice, thick chicken gravy. (Add a pinch of salt and black pepper here if need be).
3. Add the chicken gravy to the soup and mix well to combine. If you have leftover cooked rice, this is the part where you toss it in! Cover the soup with a lid and simmer for 30 minutes to let it thicken up.
4. Serve over a bowl of warm rice and enjoy!

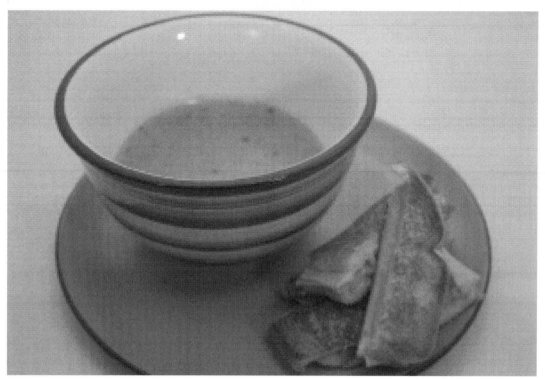

I was inspired to make my own version of this soup after tasting out at a local restaurant and not being able to get the recipe. They only serve it on Thursdays, but now we can have it any day of the week!

Thursday Pesto Tomato Soup

Serves: 4 servings

Ingredients:

- 1 large, family-size can of tomato soup (Generic or Campbell's... either is fine)
- 2 tbsp. jarred pesto
- 1 cup heavy whipping cream
- 1 tsp. garlic powder
- Salt and pepper to taste

Instructions:

1. In a large pot, pour in the can of tomato soup. Then, fill the tomato soup can halfway with water and dump it into the pot. Discard the can. Stir together until evenly combined. Turn on the stove to medium heat and bring to a simmer.
2. Once the soup begins to bubble, drop in 2 tbsp. of jarred pesto. (Try and drain off as much olive oil as possible before you drop it into the soup).

3. Next, mix the pesto through until evenly combined. Then pour in a cup of cream and mix through. Let the soup simmer for 5 minutes over medium heat.

4. Add the garlic powder, salt, and black pepper. Adjust according to your taste preferences. Serve hot and enjoy!

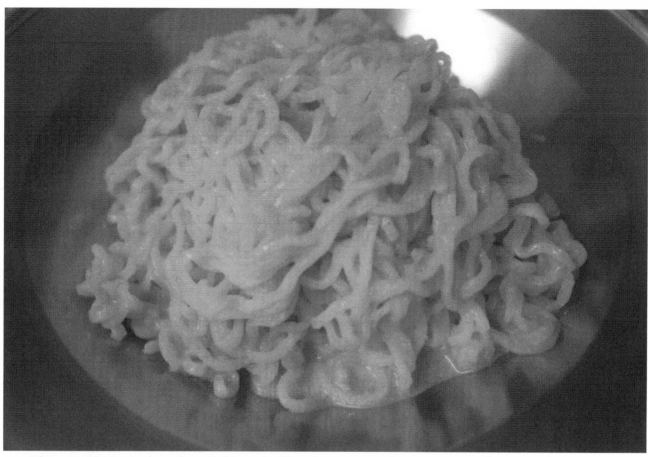

These noodz are truly unforgettable and will make you crave instant ramen all over again. Trust me.

Tasteful Noodz

Serves: 1

Ingredients:

- 1 packet of ramen chicken flavor (**Use vegan ramen if you want to adapt for veganism**)
- 3 tablespoons nutritional yeast

Instructions:

1. Gather your ingredients.
2. Bring a pot to boil with water and drop in the seasoning packet. Add the noodles and cook for 5-6 minutes.
3. Reserve 3-4 tablespoons of chicken flavored cooking water in a mixing bowl and add the noodles. Then add the nutritional yeast and mix, mix, mix!
4. Chow down and enjoy!

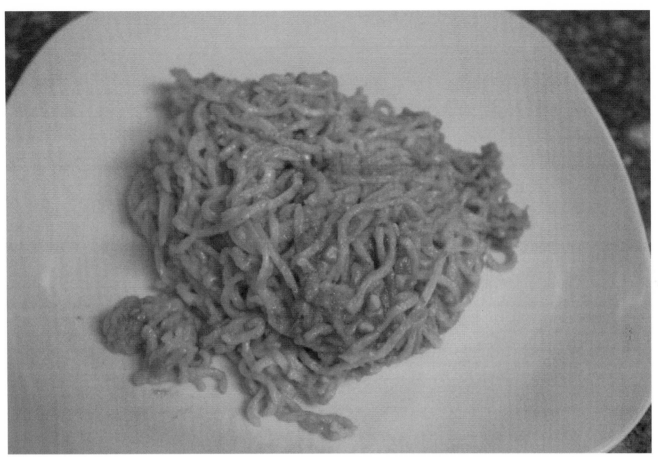

When you're in a pinch and the cupboards are bare but you're craving Thai food, let this recipe come to the rescue.

Only-Slightly-Broke Pad Thai

Serves: 1

Ingredients:

- 1 can beef broth
- 2 tablespoons chunky peanut butter
- 1 tablespoon Sriracha
- 1 teaspoon Chinese five spice
- 1 pack of ramen noodles

Instructions:

1. Gather your ingredients.
2. In a small bowl, mix up the peanut butter, sriracha, and Chinese five spice.

3. Cook your ramen noodles in the beef broth with a bit of extra water if need be. (My noodles took 5 minutes boiling). Drain and set aside.
4. Mix the sauce into the noodles carefully spreading it around as best that you can
5. Eat while hot and enjoy!

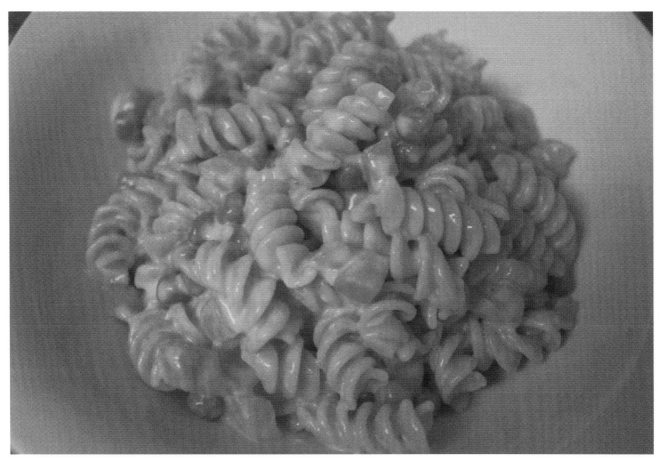

Seriously, step away from the orange powder. Once you eat this from scratch, you'll never want to go back.

Not-From-a-Box Macaroni and Cheese

Serves: 4

Ingredients:

- 1 (16 ounce) box whole wheat rotini (spiral) pasta
- 2 cups milk
- 2 cups Mexican blend cheese, or any cheese of your preference
- 2 tablespoons butter
- 1 small bag frozen peas and carrots bag (Note: We used a microwavable frozen steamer bag kind to make it easier)

Instructions:

1. Grab all of your ingredients.
2. Get a pot boiling with water and cook your spiral pasta until tender. Ours took about 10 minutes.

3. Drain the pasta. Turn the heat back on to medium-low and add in the milk, butter, and cheese. Mix, mix, mix until it's creamy and looking delicious!

4. Meanwhile microwave the frozen veggies according to the steam-bag directions. Ours took 5 minutes and was done. Add in the vegetables to the cheesy pasta. Mix and eat! Enjoy!

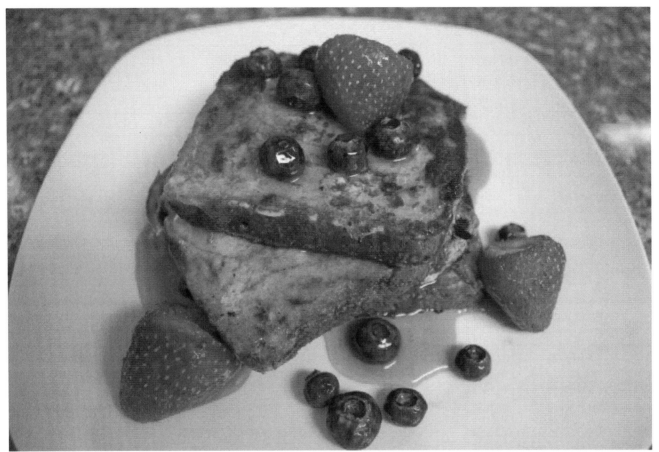

This French toast is about as simple as it gets but is sure to impress your dom or Little when you serve this for breakfast in bed.

Shortcut Cinnamon French Toast

Serves: 4

Ingredients:

- 1/2 cup milk
- 4 eggs
- 1 teaspoon vanilla extract
- 8 slices cinnamon swirl bread
- 3 tablespoons butter
- Any extra topping you'd like ▨

Instructions:

1. Gather your ingredients.
2. Crack the eggs, milk, and vanilla extract in a mixing dish. Whisk together.

3. Add the butter to a skillet and bring to medium-high heat. Dip the bread on both sides into the egg wash and place in the pan. Cook evenly until brown on both sides. (About 2-3 minutes). Repeat until all the slices are cooked.

4. Top with your favorite toppings and eat hot. Enjoy!

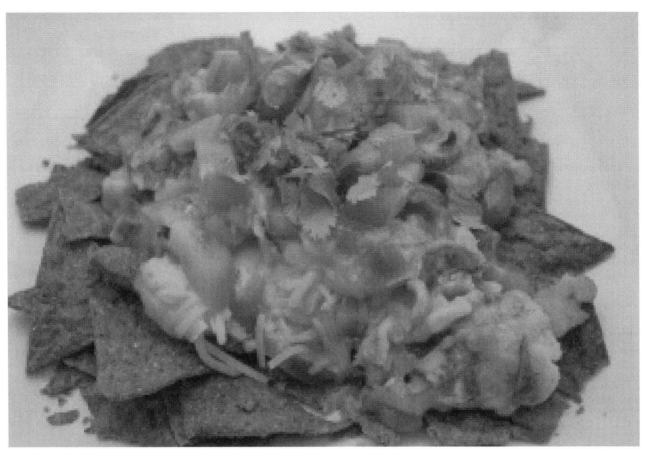

While this dish looks difficult, I promise you it is deceptively easy. In fact, your fish can go from freezer to pan without defrosting and still turn out fantastic. I pirate promise you!

Tali's Naaaaaaarchos!

Yields: 10-12 servings

Ingredients:

- 1 lb. white fish fillets (tilapia, swai, cod, etc.)
- 1 red onion, chopped
- 1 bell pepper, chopped
- 1 tomato, chopped
- 1 bunch cilantro/coriander, chopped
- 2 Yukon gold potatoes, cubed
- 1 cup Monterey Jack cheese
- 2 cups Cheddar cheese
- 1 tbsp. curry powder
- 1 tsp. garlic powder
- 1 tbsp. turmeric

- salt and pepper to taste
- drizzle of olive oil

Instructions:

1. Preheat the oven to 400 degrees (F)/ 200 degrees (C).
2. In a 9 X 13 baking dish, put in the chopped: potatoes, red onion, and bell pepper. Season thoroughly with curry powder, turmeric, garlic powder, salt, and black pepper. Mix it all around to coat everything. Take the frozen (or fresh) fish fillets and nestle them into the seasoned vegetables.
3. Then drizzle everything with a bit of olive oil. (Not so much that everything is dripping, but just enough so that it won't stick to the pan).
4. Bake for 1 hour in the oven. Then remove and while it's piping hot, sprinkle on the cheese and let stand for 2 minutes. (Don't worry... the cheese will melt!).
5. Sprinkle out nacho chips on a plate and once the cheese has melted in the pan, use a spoon to break down the fish and mix everything around. Scoop out a serving of cheesy curried nacho mix and place on top of the chips. Garnish with chopped tomatoes and cilantro and serve hot. Enjoy!

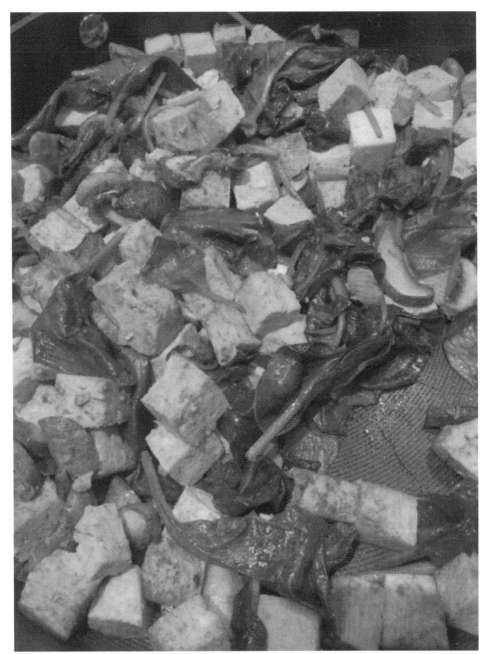

Tofu is a wonderful protein and an economical choice when you're craving Chinese takeout. This recipe will get you used to working with Tofu in a tasty simple way.

Eat Your Veg Tofu Stir-Fry

Serves: 6

Ingredients:

- 2 blocks extra firm tofu

- 1 bundle fresh spinach
- 8 ounces mushrooms, sliced
- 1/2 cup dark soy sauce
- 3 tablespoons Sriracha
- Garlic powder for seasoning

Instructions:

1. Begin by squeezing out the tofu with your hands and try to get as much water out as possible. Set aside and slice the blocks horizontally before cutting into cubes.
2. Drizzle oil in a large skillet and turn the stove on high.
3. Pop the tofu in a pan and give a generous sprinkling of garlic powder over the tofu. Use a spatula to toss it around until it gets nice and crispy (about 3-4 minutes) and just brown on the edges.
4. Next, take the Sriracha bottle and squirt a "Z" over the tofu. Then use your spatula to toss everything around again. Add the soy sauce and the mushrooms and cook until the mushrooms are tender and the liquid has evaporated. Use your spatula to continue tossing so everything gets evenly mixed in the soy sauce.
5. Finally drop in the bundle of fresh spinach and cook for an additional minute until just wilted and tender. Turn off the heat and serve over hot jasmine rice. Enjoy!

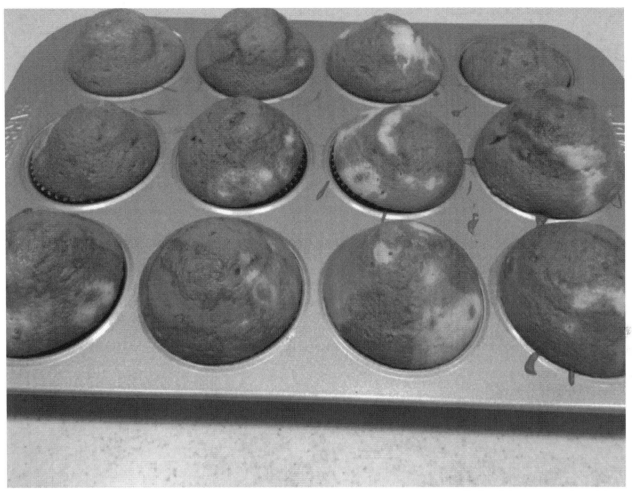

Nothing is more kawaii than a batch of rainbow cupcakes. When you need a little pick me up, give this recipe a try!

Tie Dye Cupcakes

Serves: 1 dozen

Ingredients:

- 1 box of white cake mix
- 2 eggs
- ¼ cup oil
- 1 box food coloring

Instructions:

1. In a large mixing bowl, combine the white cake mix, eggs and oil.
2. Preheat oven to 350 degrees (F)

3. Divide the batter into smaller mixing bowls.
4. Place several drops of food dye in each bowl and mix to combine.
5. Grease a muffin pan and begin spooning in different colors of the cupcake batter into each tin.
6. Fill each muffin tin approximately halfway.
7. Bake for 15 minutes or until lightly golden around edges.
8. Remove from oven and let cool completely. Then frost and serve immediately.

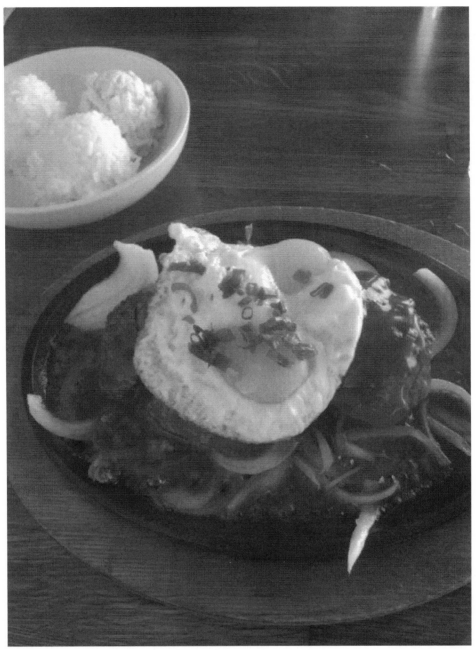

This dish is perfect for sharing together. A simple skillet of vegetables with two hamburger patties, sauce and fried eggs will leave you happily full and longing to make this again.

Loco Moco

Serves: 2

Ingredients:

- 1 onion chopped

- 1 green bell pepper chopped
- 1 lb. Ground sirloin
- 1 tablespoon ketchup
- 1 tablespoon yellow mustard
- ¼ cup of bread crumbs
- 3 eggs

For the sauce:

- 1 14 oz. can of beef broth
- 3 tablespoons of butter
- 4 tablespoons all-purpose flour

For the garnish:

- 3 green onions chopped finely

Instructions:

For the burger:

1. In a mixing bowl, combine the ground sirloin, one egg, ketchup, mustard and mix.
2. Add in bread crumbs and mix to combine. Divide into two portions and form two patties.
3. Create an indent in the center of each pattie with your thumb. Then place into a greased cooking skillet on medium high heat.
4. Cover and cook for four minutes on one side. Flip the burgers over and continue cooking for additional four minutes. Remove and set aside.

For the skillet:

1. In the greased skillet, place the onion and green bell pepper. Sauté for five to seven minutes on medium-high heat or until tender.
2. Remove and set aside.

For the sauce:

1. In a small cooking pan, over medium heat, melt the butter. Add the flour and mix to create a roux.
2. Add the can of beef broth and continue stirring until it begins to thicken into a gravy.
3. Season with salt and pepper as needed then set aside.

For the garnish:

1. In the greased skillet, fry two eggs sunny side up (2–3 minutes).
2. While the eggs are frying, chop several green onions for garnish.
3. To plate, place the sautéed vegetables on the bottom, place the burger patties on top. Drizzle both patties generously with the sauce. Top with fried eggs and green onions and serve while hot.

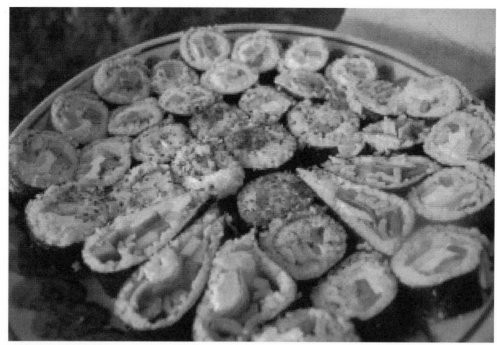

Daddy's sushi platter is a reward for every good Little. While this dish looks complicated, if you help prep in the kitchen — it quickly becomes a breeze.

Daddy's Sushi

Serves: 4

Recommended Ingredients:

- 2 cups jasmine rice
- 1 tablespoon rice vinegar
- 4 sheets nori seaweed
- 1 cucumber, julienned
- 1 pickled daikon radish, julienned
- 1 pack imitation crab, sliced
- 1 pack dried fish cake
- 4 slices cooked spam
- 1 carrot, julienned

Instructions:

1. Prepare the rice by adding a few splashes of rice vinegar into the rice cooker with the jasmine rice and water.
2. Get a bamboo mat (or cheap, flexible placemat) and place a sheet of Nori Seaweed on it. Take a spoon and gently press cooked jasmine rice onto the seaweed.

3. Slice all of your seafood and produce in long thin strips. Don't worry about knife cuts here. Just make sure they are relatively thin so you are able to roll everything up easier.
4. Lay your sushi roll ingredients at the edge of the rice and seaweed.
5. Using the mat, carefully roll and tuck the seaweed over the ingredients and continue to gently roll up your sushi. If you need to stop and gently tuck in bits of rice, that's fine. Go slow and steady to ensure that nothing rips or falls out.
6. Use a sharp knife to cut your sushi into thin rounds. Set everything on a platter and enjoy! Note: I also served this with a jar of pickled ginger (available in most Asian markets for $2 USD), and soy sauce for dipping.

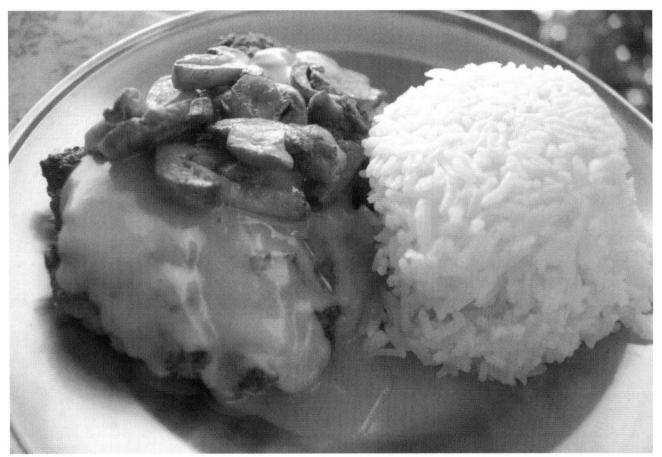

East meets West in this Southern fusion dish. This easy Salisbury steak can be paired with rice or pasta for a filling weeknight meal.

Easy Salisbury Steak

Serves: 6

Ingredients:

For the burgers:

- 2 lbs. ground beef
- 4 tbsp. ketchup
- 1 tbsp. yellow mustard
- 2 tbsp. soy sauce
- 1 tbsp. garlic powder
- 1 tsp. Worcestershire Sauce
- 1 onion, diced
- 1/2 cup bread crumbs
- Salt and black pepper to taste

For the Gravy:

- 1/4 c. or 1/2 stick of butter
- 1/4 c. flour
- 2 cups (or 1- 14.5 ounce can) beef broth
- 1 pack mushrooms, sautéed
- Vegetable oil for frying

Instructions:

1. Pour a bit of oil in the pan. Drop in mushroom slices. Sauté for 5-10 minutes or until tender. Set aside in a bowl.
2. In a large mixing bowl, combine all ingredients for hamburgers except bread crumbs. Mix well to combine. Then add bread crumbs and mix to form patties.
3. Make an indention in the center of each patty with your thumb.
4. Pour oil in a deep-frying pan and heat on medium-high heat.
5. Drop in 2 patties at a time and fry for 3 minutes. Flip over and fry on the other side for 3 more minutes. Set aside on a plate to cool. Repeat until all patties are cooked.
6. Now it's time to make the gravy! In a pot, add the butter over medium heat and let melt. Then add in the flour and whisk to make a roux.
7. Next, pour in the beef broth and mix slowly to combine. Add a pinch of salt and a few dashes of black pepper. Continue to mix until the gravy has thickened.
8. To plate: Place 1 cup of steamed rice on the plate. Add 2 burger patties. Top the burgers with beef gravy and garnish with sautéed mushrooms. Serve hot and enjoy!

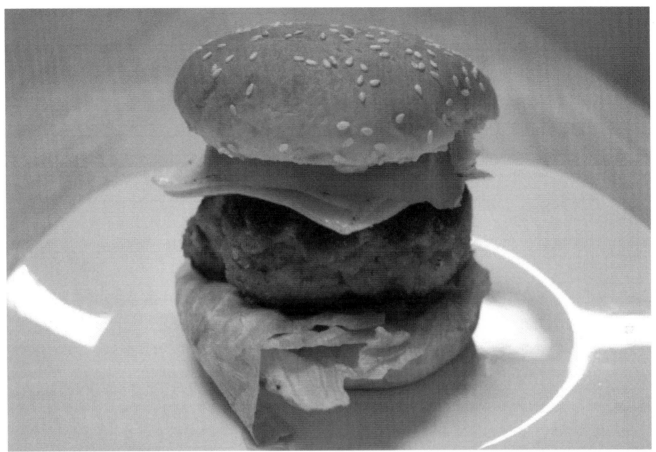

This cheeseburger recipe is perfect for you and your Little one an American diner night at home. Pair this with a bag of french fries or onion rings and you're ready to go. Bonus points if you make homemade milkshakes.

Diner Cheeseburgers

Serves: 4 burgers

Ingredients:

- 1.5 lbs. extra lean ground turkey
- 1 egg, lightly beaten
- 1/2 teaspoon salt
- 1/2 teaspoon pepper
- 1 tablespoon olive oil
- 4 sesame seed hamburger buns
- Toppings of your choice

Instructions:

1. In a large bowl, combine bread crumbs, egg, salt and pepper. Add beef; mix lightly but thoroughly. Shape into four 1/2-in.-thick patties. Press a shallow indentation in the center of each with your thumb. Brush both sides of patties with oil.

2. Grill burgers, covered, over medium heat or broil 4 in. from heat 4-5 minutes on each side or until a thermometer reads 160°. Serve on buns with toppings and enjoy!

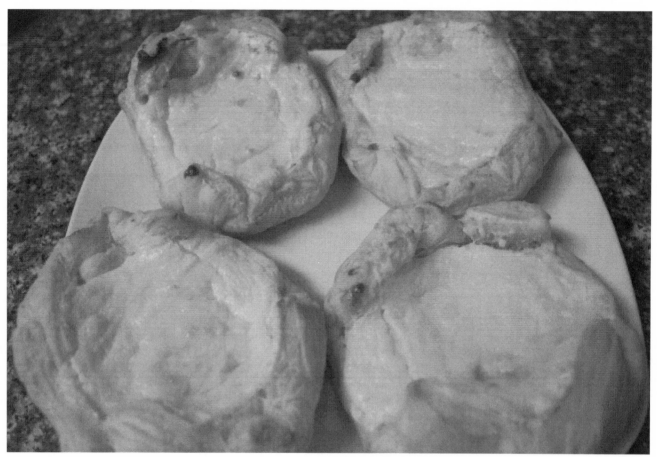

Bring the patisserie home with these simple homemade cheese Danish. You and your Little one will swoon over the buttery, flaky taste in these treats.

Homemade Cheese Danish

Serves: 8 Danish

Ingredients:

- 2 sheets puff pastry, thawed but cool
- 1 (8 ounce) block cream cheese, at room temperature
- 1/2 cup sugar
- 1 tsp. vanilla extract

- 2 eggs, divided
- A bit of flour for rolling out the puff pastry

Instructions:

1. First preheat your oven to 400 degrees F/ 204 C. Then in two small bowls separate your egg yolks and whites. Set aside.
2. Next, make your Danish filling! In a stand mixer cream together the cream cheese, sugar, vanilla extract, and 2 egg yolks. Mmmm creamy! ⊠
3. Meanwhile roll out your puff pastry sheets on a floured area to about 10 x 10 and divide into 4 squares.
4. Take a tablespoon of filling (go generous here!) and place in the center of each square.
5. Brush the edges of each Danish with egg white and then crimp up the sides and corners of each Danish until they are just touching the cheese filling.
6. Bake in a preheated oven at 400 degrees F/ 204 degrees C for 10 minutes. Then rotate your pan and bake for another 10 minutes until it's golden brown. Serve hot and enjoy!

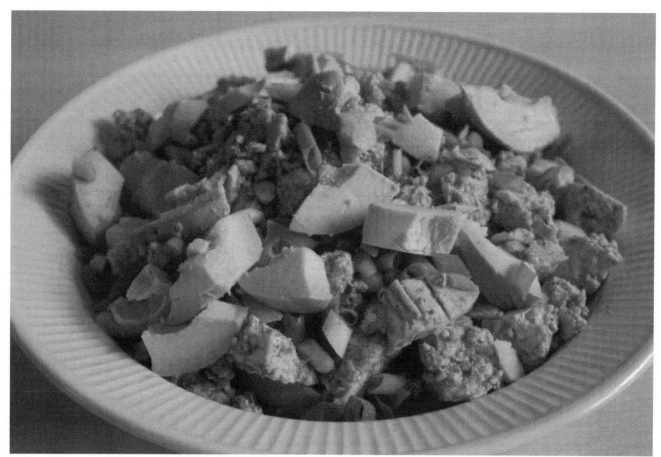

This Sofritas bowl is perfect for cooking with your sub because it takes a bland block of tofu and transforms it into a delicious Mexican meal. Purrrfect for when you're feeling lazy and don't want to cook!

Lazy Cat Sofritas Bowl

Serves: 6-8 servings

Ingredients:

- 1 can black beans, drained and heated
- 1 can corn drained
- 1 tomato, diced
- 3 green onions, diced
- 1 avocado, peeled and diced

For Sofritas Tofu:

- 1 block extra firm tofu
- 2 tsp. salt
- 1 tsp. red chili pepper powder (I used Korean Gochugaru)

- 1 tsp. ground coriander
- 1 tsp. ground cumin
- 1 tsp. Sriracha
- 1 tsp. minced ginger
- 1 tsp. minced garlic
- 1 tbsp. rice wine vinegar
- 1 tbsp. canola oil

Instructions:

1. In a large skillet, pour oil in the pan and turn on the stove to medium heat. Drain and crumble the tofu in your hands and drop into the pan. Wait until the tofu begins to sizzle.
2. Then add the salt, vinegar, garlic, ginger, and all of the spices and mix through the tofu until well combined. Let the tofu continue cooking on medium-high heat for 2-3 minutes. Then add the Sriracha and fry for an additional minute. At this point the tofu should be crispy on the edges.
3. In a microwave safe bowl, drain and heat up the can for black beans for about 1 min. 30 seconds. Then pour into a communal bowl.
4. Top with a can of corn (drained), diced tomatoes, and then add the tofu on top.
5. Garnish with green onions and diced avocado. Serve hot with tortilla chips and enjoy!

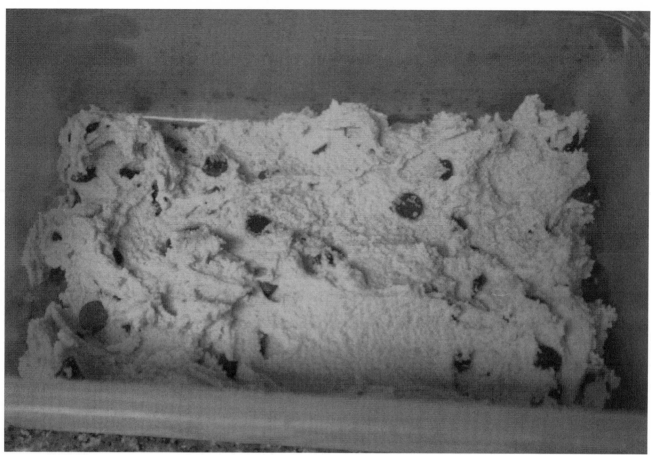

Every Little girl needs a recipe for chocolate chip cookies. But eating cookie dough raw can be dangerous. That's why my Daddy created this recipe to keep in the freezer and nibble any time you need a Little treat.

Daddy's Freezer Cookie Dough

Serves: About 2 cups

Ingredients:

- 8 tablespoons Earth Balance Spread
- 3/4 cup brown sugar
- 1 teaspoon vanilla extract
- 1/2 teaspoon salt
- 1 cup all-purpose flour
- 2 tablespoons almond milk
- 1/2 cup vegan chocolate chips

Instructions:

1. Cream the vegan butter and sugar together in a stand mixer.
2. Add in the vanilla extract and salt. Mix until well combined.
3. Next add in the flour and almond milk and mix well.
4. Finally add in the chocolate chips. Pour into a freezer-friendly food storage and freeze for at least 4 hours. Enjoy!

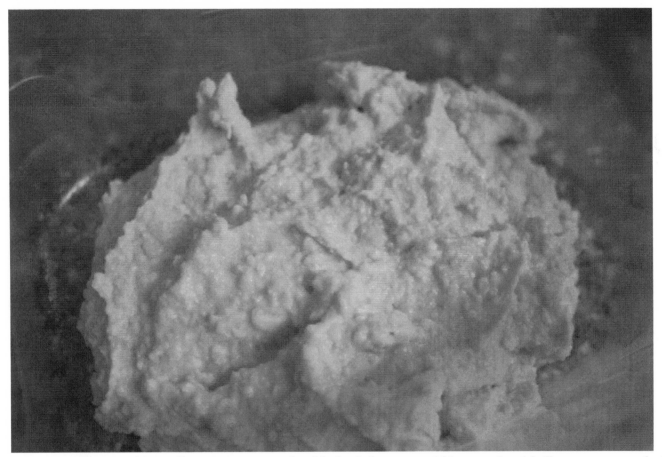

With just a couple of ingredients, you can make this basic hummus. Add roasted red bell peppers or cooked beets or Vegan pesto to take this to the next level.

Easy Hummus Dip

Serves: 2

Ingredients:

- 1 can of chickpeas
- 2 tbsp. olive oil
- 1/4 cup lemon juice
- 1/4 cup tahini

- 1 clove garlic
- 1/2 tsp. salt
- 1/4 tsp. ground cumin

Instructions:

1. Drain the chickpeas and put into a food processor. Add everything else and puree until smooth and creamy. (Add an extra tablespoon of olive oil if need be).
2. Place into a Tupperware and chill until you're ready to serve. Enjoy!

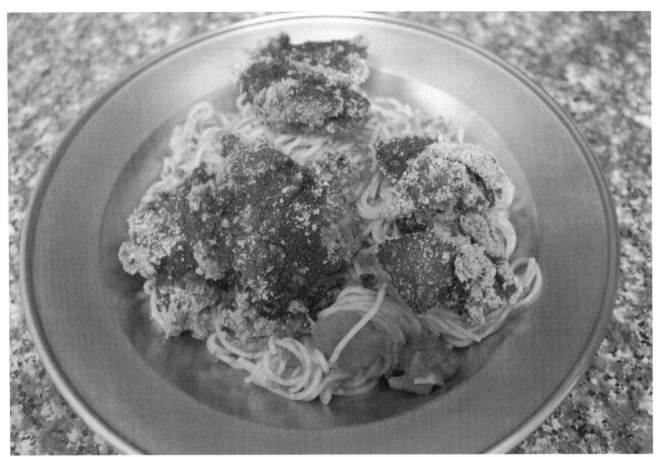

If you like Chicken Parmesan, you'll love this spin on simple spaghetti. Oven-baked livers are a budget friendly and tasty option in place of chicken nuggets. (They are a great source of iron too!)

Oven Baked Livers

Serves: 12-15 baked livers

Ingredients:

- 2 (1 lb.) tubs of chicken livers
- 1 stick butter, melted
- 2 cups Italian Breadcrumbs

Instructions:

1. Preheat the oven to 350 degrees (F)/ 180 degrees (C).
2. Rinse the livers in a small colander. Then set aside in a bowl.
3. Pour the melted butter in a bowl. Then pour the breadcrumbs in a separate bowl. Now you have three bowls in a row: one with liver, one with butter, and one with breadcrumbs. Now time to dip!

4. Dip the livers in butter, then coat with breadcrumbs, then place on a greased baking sheet. Repeat until all the livers are coated.
5. Bake for 45 minutes in the oven. Then set aside to rest. Top on spaghetti and chow down!

Simple Spaghetti

Serves: 6 portions

Ingredients:

- 1 box angel hair pasta
- 1 jar pasta sauce

Instructions:

1. Boil the angel hair for 7 minutes. Drain and dump back into the pot.
2. Toss in the sauce over the hot noodles and mix well to combine.
3. Serve into portions and top with oven baked livers. Chow down!!

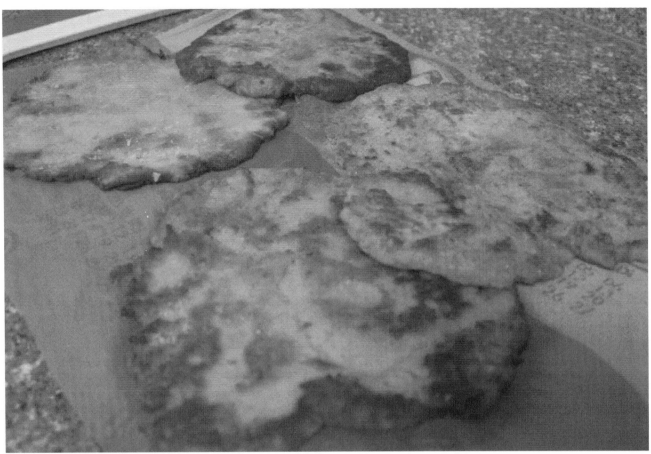

These flatbreads require only three ingredients and keep the pure, unrefined flavor of sweet potato. They are perfect to pair with falafel, chicken, or any type of wrap.

Sweet Potato Flatbread

Serves: 4

Ingredients:

- 2 Yams, peeled, boiled, and mashed
- 1 tsp. salt
- 1 cup all-purpose flour + 1/2 cup for dusting and kneading

Instructions:

1. Peel and then boil the sweet potatoes until tender. Around 20 minutes.
2. Drain and set in a bowl to mash. Mash until smooth.
3. Add the salt and mix into the potatoes.
4. Then add 1 cup of flour into the potatoes and mix until it forms a loose, crumbly dough.

5. Pour 1/2 cup of flour onto your counter. Grab a handful of sweet potato dough and mix into the flour on your counter. Knead until it forms a loose dough. Then roll out to desired thinness.
6. Heat a skillet to medium-high heat with enough vegetable oil to cover the bottom.
7. Fry bread on each side until golden-dark. 1-2 minutes per side. Set aside to cool. Serve hot with toppings such as: falafel, sabich, etc.

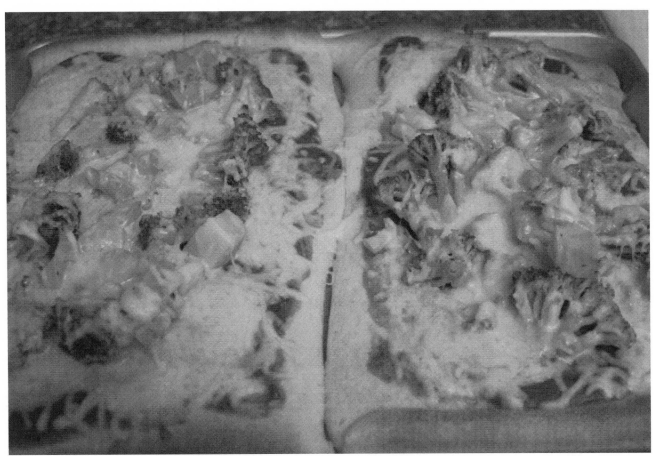

This pizza is perfect for sneaking in some vegetables while still letting the broccoli shine. You'll be surprised at how delicious and easy this pizza recipe is.

Green Pizza

Serves: 6

Ingredients:

- 3 cans pre-made pizza dough
- 1 jar marinara sauce
- 1 jar pesto
- 1 small bag frozen broccoli
- 3 cups low-fat Mozzarella cheese

Instructions:

1. Preheat your oven to 450 degrees (F)/ 230 degrees (C).

2. Grease two baking sheets and roll out the dough on the pan. While the oven is warming up, fill a pot with water and drop in the broccoli. Boil for 10-15 minutes or until tender when pricked with a fork. Drain and set aside.

3. When the oven is preheated, slip in your dough. Bake for 8 minutes on a middle rack.

4. Remove from oven. Top with several tablespoons of marinara sauce and pesto (to your liking). Add the cooked broccoli. Then top with cheese.

5. Bake for an additional 8 minutes until the pizza is just turning golden around the edges. And you're done! Serve hot and enjoy!

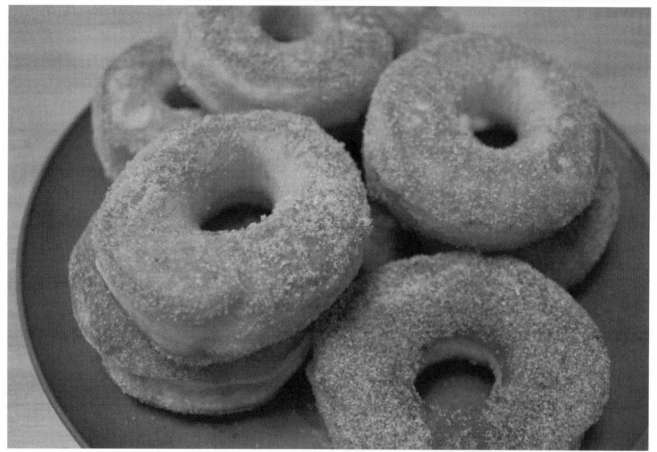

I don't know about you, but I LOVE donuts! With this two-ingredient recipe, you can make all kinds of donuts, such as: cinnamon sugar, powdered sugar, chocolate frosted, glazed, etc.

Two-Ingredient Donuts

Serves: 8 doughnuts

Ingredients:

- 1 (8 count) can buttermilk biscuit dough
- Vegetable oil for frying

- Any toppings you desire!

Instructions:

1. Begin by placing a skillet on medium heat to warm with enough vegetable oil to fry your donuts.
2. While the skillet is warming, open the can of biscuit dough. Use a donut cutter, or a shot glass, to cut out a hole in your donuts. Save the holes to make doughnut holes!
3. Once the oil is hot, gently place your donuts in 3-4 at a time. Fry on each side for 3-4 minutes or until golden brown. Flip and fry on the other side for the same amount of time. Continue frying until all of your donuts and donut holes are cooked.
4. Remove from the pan onto a towel-lined plate. Then dip your donuts into your preferred topping.
5. Serve hot and enjoy!

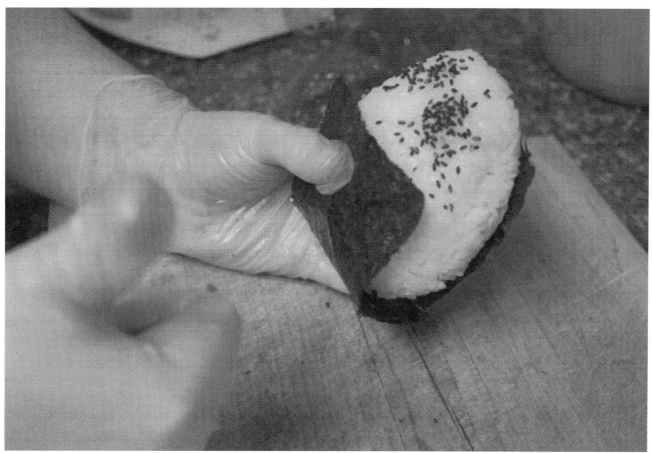

I felt so proud when I made these Vegan onigiri and I know you will too. I prefer my filling to be mushroom and greens, but you can easily adapt your own flavors into this rice ball on the go.

Vegan Onigiri

Serves: 4

Ingredients:

- 2 cups cooked rice
- 3 teaspoons rice wine vinegar
- 4 tablespoons soy sauce
- 1 tablespoon garlic powder
- 2 cups sliced mushrooms
- 2 cups fresh baby spinach
- oil for frying

Instructions:

1. Begin by cooking your rice. In my rice cooker I usually prepare 2 cups of rice with 3.5 cups of water and it takes around 40m for the rice cooker to steam it up.
2. While your rice is cooking, go ahead and sauté your mushrooms and spinach in a small pan. Put the veg in a medium-high saucepan and pour in 3-4 tbsp. of soy sauce and a pinch of garlic powder. Cook until soft and tender then remove and set aside.
3. Once the rice is cooked I lay out a piece of plastic wrap on a sturdy surface. Then I spoon the rice into a mixing bowl and put 3 teaspoons of rice wine vinegar into it. I mix it all up and I'm ready to begin assembling the onigiri!
4. First begin by spooning about 1 cup of cooked rice into the plastic wrap. If you have plastic gloves, wet them just a little and press the rice down into a circle. If not, use the back of a wet spoon and press the rice down. Then make a small indention in the middle.
5. Place some chopped, cooked veggies in the center of the rice.
6. Carefully start grabbing the ends of the plastic wrap to create a little bundle in your hands.
7. Then start twisting the onigiri around and around in your hand. As you're tightening the sack, gently shape the sticky rice into a ball to hold everything inside. And then you have a ball!
8. Now gently shape the ball into a triangle and wrap it in a piece of Nori seaweed.
9. Sprinkle with furikake seasoning and you're ready to eat! Mmmm! Smell that seaweed being heated up by the hot rice. So delicious!!

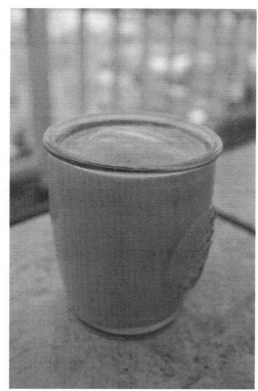

This Very Berry Smoothie is perfect for breakfast on the go. Pour this into your kawaii sippy cup and you're sure to be the envy of all your friends.

Very Berry Morning Smoothie

Serves: 2 generously

Ingredients:

- 1 cup soy milk
- 1/2 cup rolled oats
- 1 banana, broken into pieces
- 14 frozen strawberries
- 1/2 teaspoon vanilla extract
- 1 1/2 teaspoons white sugar

Instructions:

1. In a blender, combine everything and blend until smooth. Pour into glasses and serve immediately. Enjoy!

My Daddy knows that when it comes to a rough day anything with Christmas is sure to make me smile. These chocolate gingerbread cookies are subtly sweet with that gingery bite that you are looking for. I know you'll enjoy them as much as I do.

Daddy's Chocolate Gingerbread Cookies

Serves: 2 dozen Gingerbread Cookies

Ingredients:

- 1/2 cup butter, softened
- 3/4 cup sugar
- 1 egg
- 1/2 cup molasses
- 3 cups all-purpose flour
- 2 tablespoons plus 1-1/2 teaspoons baking cocoa
- 1 teaspoon baking soda
- 1 teaspoon ground cinnamon
- 1 teaspoon ground ginger
- 1/2 teaspoon ground cardamom

- 1/2 teaspoon ground nutmeg
- 1/4 teaspoon ground garam masala
- 1/2 teaspoon baking powder
- 1/2 teaspoon salt

Instructions:

1. First cream the butter and sugar together in a bowl. Then beat in the egg and molasses.
2. Combine the dry ingredients: flour, cocoa, baking soda, cinnamon, baking powder, salt, and spices.
3. Add the dry ingredients to the wet ingredients and mix until thoroughly combined.
4. Cover and refrigerate for 1 hour.
5. Preheat the oven to 350 degrees (F). Roll out the dough to about a 1/8-inch thickness.
6. Cut the dough into little (or big) gingerbread people.
7. Place on a greased cookie sheet and bake for 8 minutes for until the edges are firm.
8. Place on a wire rack to cool, then decorate, and enjoy!

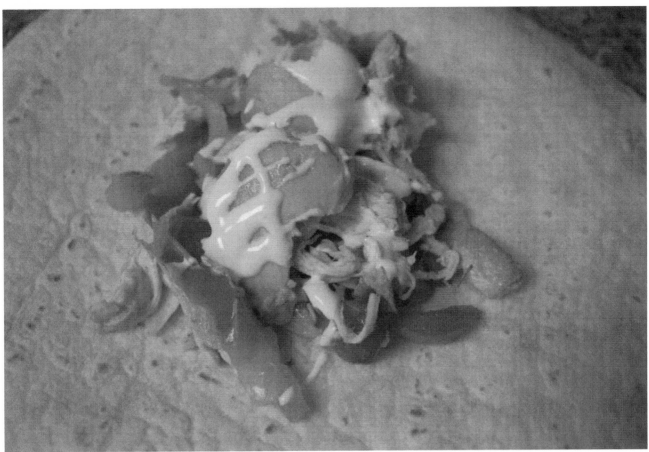

These five ingredient fajitas are so simple to make that any Little can do it. Make these for your dom the next time you want Taco Tuesday.

Five Ingredient Fajitas

Serves: 4 servings

Ingredients:

- 1 cooked chicken breast, shredded
- 1 avocado, peeled and mashed
- 1 bag frozen bell pepper strips
- 2 tbsp. Mexican Crema
- 1 package taco tortillas (Note: I had burrito tortillas on hand in this pic. But if you're buying supplies, go for the smaller ones.)
- Cajun seasoning (optional)

Instructions:

1. First gather your ingredients.
2. Then, toss a bit of oil and the frozen peppers in a pan.
3. Once they are cooked, toss in the chicken and cook until warmed through.
4. Use Cajun seasoning to give things a kick.
5. Peel your avocado. Mmmm.... Avocado!
6. Slap the filling in a tortilla. Top with avocado. Drizzle on the crema and shove that baby in your face! YUM!!! Enjoy everyone!

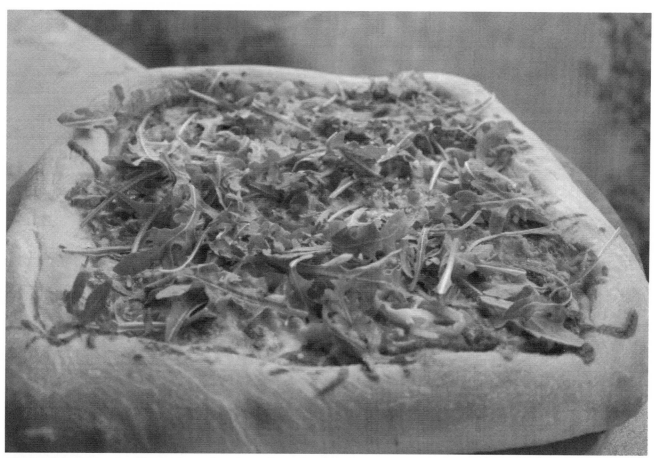

This Italian style pizza looks fancy but is really quite simple to make. Get your fingers messy making the dough and then let your imagination run wild with the toppings.

Italian Pizza

Serves: 4 servings

Ingredients:

For the Dough:

- 2 1/4 cups flour
- 1 teaspoon salt
- 1 teaspoon yeast
- 1 teaspoon honey
- 1 cup warm water

For the Pizza:

- 6 slices Italian Salami, diced
- 1 cup jarred banana pepper slices, drained
- 1 cup fresh arugula
- 1/3 cup pizza sauce
- 1 cup Mozzarella Cheese
- 2 tablespoons olive oil

Instructions:

1. If you have a bread machine: place the flour and salt inside the machine canister. In a separate bowl, add the warm water and honey. Mix to combine. Add the yeast and set in a warm place for 3 minutes to activate the yeast. (It should bubble). Then add the yeast mixture into the flour and close the bread machine. Set the machine to the "Dough" setting and let it go for 1.5 hours.

2. If you don't have a bread machine: Begin by placing the flour and salt in a large, greased mixing bowl. Activate the yeast in a separate mixing bowl by adding 1 cup of warm water and 1 teaspoon of honey mixed. Add the yeast into the honey water and set in a warm spot for 3 minutes. (It should bubble). Then pour into the flour and mix until well combined, or use a stand mixer with a dough hook attachment. Cover the dough in the bowl with plastic wrap to form a seal. Place in a warm, draft-free spot and cover the bowl with a kitchen towel. Let rise for 1 hour.

3. Then punch down and knead the dough on a floured surface for 5 minutes. Place back into the mixing bowl. Re-seal with plastic wrap and a kitchen towel and let it rise again for an additional hour. Then the dough is ready to use!

4. Now prepare the pizza. Roll out the dough to a 1-1/2 inch thickness. Pour 2 tablespoons of olive oil on the dough and brush all around the pizza.

5. Make an indention 1/2 inch from the outer perimeter of the pizza with your finger and use your other hand to create a raised edge on the outside of the pizza. This will create a fluffy ring to hold your sauce and toppings inside the pizza.

6. Next spread the sauce on the pizza. Then add the diced salami, banana peppers, and cheese.

7. Bake at 450 degrees (F)/ 230 degrees (C) for 20-25 minutes. Remove and top with fresh arugula. Serve hot and enjoy!

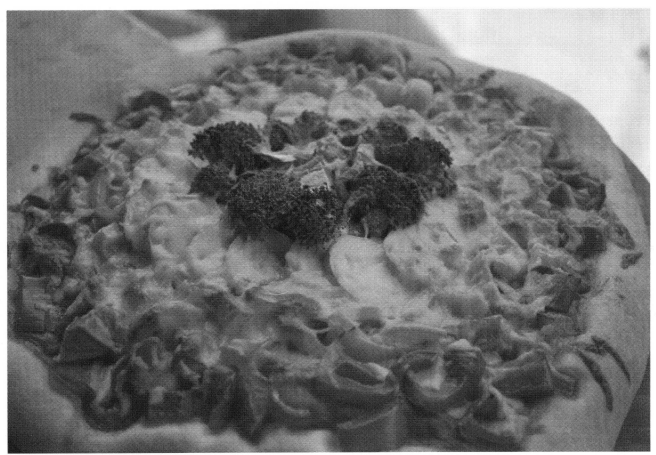

This pizza looks elegant while still letting you get your five a day. Eating your vegetables has never tasted better.

Rainbow Pizza

Serves: 6-8 servings

Ingredients:

- 1 red bell pepper, diced
- 1 orange bell pepper, diced
- 2 small yellow squash, cut into rings
- 1 cup broccoli florets
- 1/4 cup purple onion, peeled and diced
- 1/3 cup pizza sauce
- 1/2 cup Mozzarella cheese
- 1 14-inch pizza pie (see previous recipe for dough)

Instructions:

1. In a skillet, sauté the bell peppers until slightly softened, about 8-10 minutes over medium heat. Set aside in a bowl. Then add the onion to the pan and sauté for 3-4 minutes until slightly softened and set aside in a separate bowl.
2. Preheat the oven to 450 degrees (F).
3. If you're using homemade dough, roll out the dough on a lightly floured surface to make a 14-inch pizza pie. Create an indention about 1/2-inch from the edge of the pizza, and use your other hand to make a raised edge on the outside of the pizza.
4. Spread the sauce on the pizza carefully with a tablespoon and smooth it out across the pizza. Then begin assembling your rainbow. Place the red bell peppers along the edge of the pizza sauce. Then add the orange bell pepper pieces. Next, add the yellow summer squash circles taking care to make them look uniform on the pizza. Next add the broccoli florets. Finally place diced purple onion pieces in the center of the pizza.
5. Top with 1/2 cup of Mozzarella cheese and bake for 20-25 minutes. Serve hot and enjoy!

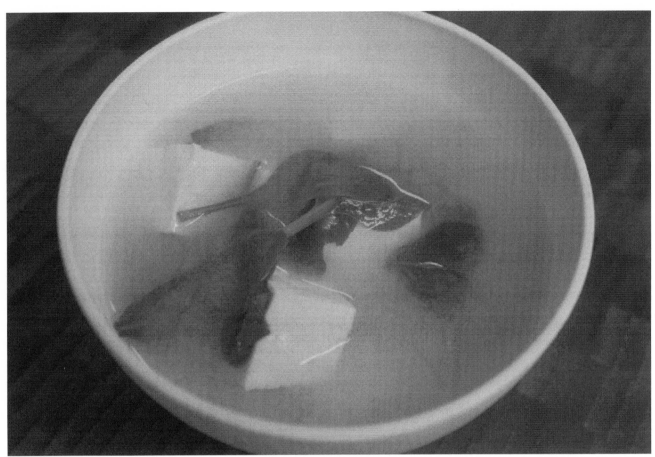

Miso soup is clean, refreshing and full of vitamins and minerals that we all need. It is wonderful when fighting a cold or if you just want a hot breakfast.

Easy Miso Soup

Serves: 6-8 servings

Ingredients:

- 1 tsp. dashi granules
- 4 cups water
- 1 block tofu, drained and cubed
- 1 handful wakame (dried seaweed) *
- 1 tablespoon miso paste

Instructions:

1. In a soup pot, bring 4 cups of water to a simmer. Add in 1 teaspoon of dashi granules. Mix to combine.
2. Then add the dried seaweed. Let it simmer for 3-4 minutes or until it fluffs up.

3. Slowly drop in the tofu and let it simmer just until warmed through.
4. Using a fine strainer, place the tablespoon of miso paste on the strainer and dip it into the broth and mix to loosen the miso paste to slowly release into the soup. (This will also protect the tofu from breaking apart so you're not mixing throughout the pot).
5. Ladle into bowls and eat hot. Enjoy!

Note: you can substitute wakame for fresh baby spinach if you can't get a hold of any.

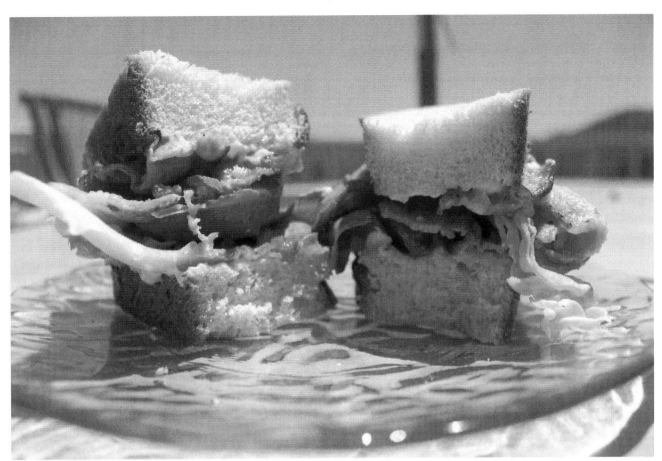

My grandma taught me how scrumptious a lettuce, tomato and mayonnaise sandwich is. I added bacon to mine and put it on two slices of challah bread. I know you'll love it too.

Gammie's LTMB Sandwich

Serves: 1

Ingredients:

- 2 pieces of lettuce
- 1 slice of tomato
- 2 strips of bacon
- 2 tablespoons mayonnaise
- 2 slices of challah bread

Instructions:

1. Slather the mayonnaise on the bread.
2. Assemble ingredients. Enjoy!

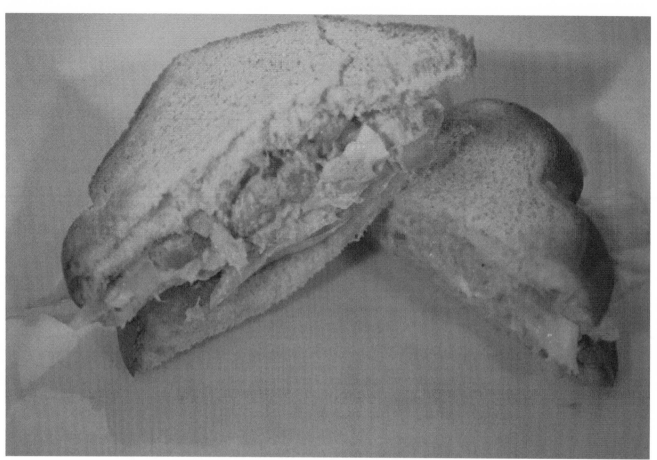

Sandwiches are a Little's perfect recipe in the kitchen. Why? Because you can play around with so many combinations and ingredients. The addition of sweet corn in the sandwich gives the tuna salad a big lift.

Tuna, Corn, and Celery Sandwich

Serves: 6 sandwiches

Ingredients:

- 3 cans of tuna, drained
- 1 can of corn, drained
- 3 ribs of celery, rinsed and chopped
- 4 tablespoons of mayonnaise
- 2 hard-boiled eggs, peeled and mashed (optional)
- 12 slices of bread, toasted
- Salt and black pepper to taste

Instructions:

1. In a large mixing bowl, add the tuna, corn, chopped celery. Mix to combine. Fold in the mayonnaise taking care to not over-mix.

2. Add in the mashed hard-boiled eggs and fold through. Season with salt and pepper according to your preference.

3. Toast your bread and place 2 tbsp. of filling on each sandwich. (I like to add chopped lettuce to mine too). Cut in half and serve immediately. Chill remaining filling. Enjoy!

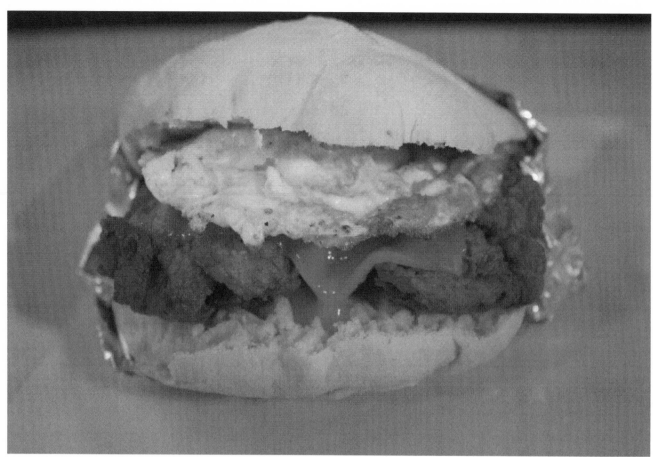

As a kitten from the deep South of the United States, fried chicken is a breakfast food where I come from. This is my recreation of a childhood breakfast sandwich that I used to eat so long ago.

Chicken, Egg, and Cheese Biscuits

Serves: 4 Breakfast Sandwiches

Ingredients:

- 4 (6-inch) rounds of homemade biscuit dough
- 4 eggs, fried
- 4 slices of Cheddar cheese

For Fried Chicken:

- 1 1/2 lbs. boneless chicken thighs
- 3 eggs
- 1/3 cup water
- 1 cup hot sauce
- 2 cups self-rising flour

- 2 tablespoons garlic powder
- Salt and black pepper to taste

Instructions:

1. Begin by making the biscuit dough a few hours beforehand. Wrap it in aluminum to chill. When you're ready to bake, preheat the oven to 425 degrees (F)/ 220 degrees (C). Place the biscuit rounds on a greased baking sheet and bake for 15 minutes, or until the tops are just golden.
2. While the biscuits are baking, fry your chicken. Line up mixing bowls in an assembly line. In the first bowl whisk together 3 eggs, 1/3 cup of water, and 1 cup of hot sauce. (The mixture should look bright orange). Next fill another mixing bowl with the flour. In a mixing bowl, rinse your chicken. Then season with salt, pepper, and garlic powder.
3. Fill a deep fryer or deep pot with vegetable oil enough so the chicken can be fully submerged. Heat to 350 degrees over high heat.
4. Dip each thigh into egg, then flour, and then use tongs to carefully drop it into the hot oil. Fry the thighs for 8-10 minutes each. Set aside on a plate.
5. As soon as you set the thigh aside, place a slice of cheese on top so it can begin to melt over it.
6. Grab a skillet and cook up eggs your favorite way. Preferably you want to have non-runny yolks, so fried eggs or scrambled are best. But do what works best for you!
7. As soon as the biscuits are done baking, pop them out of the oven and set aside to cool for 5 minutes. Then slice in half. Place a piece of chicken on the biscuit, followed by an egg. Top with the biscuit top. Serve hot and enjoy!

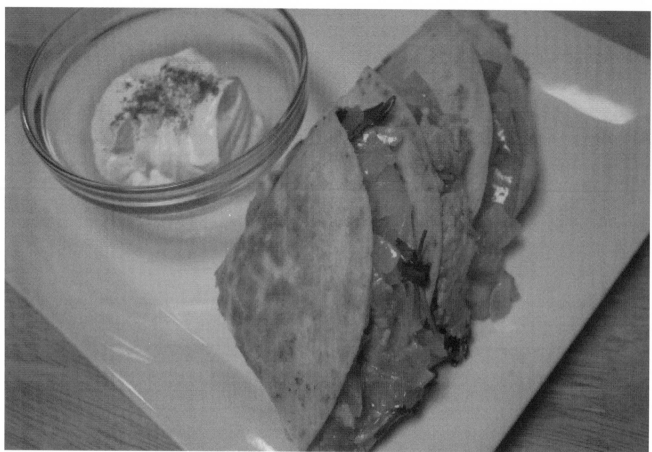

Quesadillas are the perfect food or appetizer when you need to use up leftover vegetables in your crisper. Add avocado to bring a creamy element to your quesadilla and make sure to toast the tortillas to create perfection.

Budget Quesadillas

Serves: 4 quesadillas

Ingredients:

- 4 tortillas
- 2 tbsp oil (I used coconut oil)
- 1 onion, peeled and diced
- 1 avocado, mashed
- 1 tomato, chopped
- 1/2 bunch cilantro, chopped
- 2 cups shredded Cheddar cheese

Instructions:

1. Grab a deep skillet and drizzle in the oil. Heat the pan over medium-high heat.
2. Drop in the tortilla. Then immediately put down a sprinkle of cheese.
3. Add your toppings and place a handful of cheese on top. Let the tortilla fry for 30 seconds longer.
4. Use a spatula to fold the tortilla in half, (like an omelet), and continue cooking for 30 seconds longer to melt the cheese.
5. Remove from pan. Cut into quarter triangles and serve hot. Enjoy!

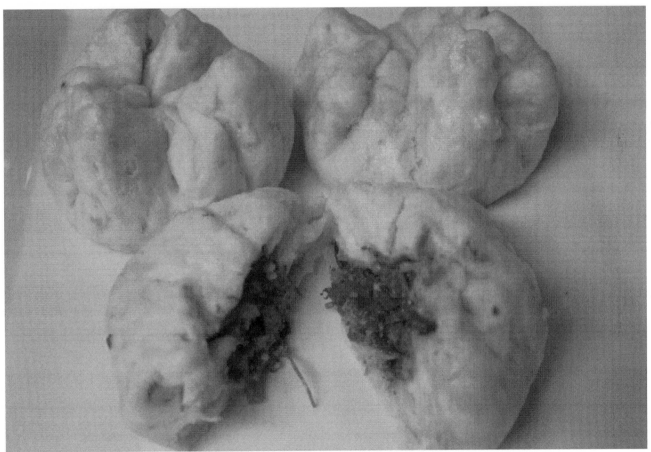

These shortcut dim sum allow you to have these Chinese street foods without all the work. Using canned biscuit dough, these dim sums can be modified for meat eaters and vegans alike.

Shortcut Dim Sum

Serves: 16 buns

Ingredients:

For the Dough:

- 2 (8-count) cans of biscuit dough

For Filling:

- 2 tablespoons minced garlic
- 1 tablespoon minced ginger
- 2 tablespoons soy sauce
- 2 tablespoons sweet chili sauce
- 2 tablespoons rice wine vinegar
- 2 packages (or 450 grams) mixed mushrooms
- 1/2 bunch of cilantros, leaves removed and stalks diced
- 4 green onions, chopped

Instructions:

1. Begin by filling up water in your steamer pot and get it heating up over high heat.
2. Now it's time to make the filling! Grab a large skillet and put in the minced garlic and ginger with a tiny drizzle of oil. Heat for 30 seconds on high heat. Add the cilantro stalks and cook for 1-2 minutes or until just softened.
3. Pulse the mushrooms in a food processor to dice, or chop finely. Then add to the skillet and cook for 4-5 minutes until softened.
4. Add the soy sauce, vinegar, and sweet chili and mix well.
5. Use a fine strainer to drain the mixture completely. Get as much liquid out of it as you can!
6. Then set the mushroom filling aside. Open the biscuit dough and, on a floured surface, roll each biscuit out just slightly to the palm of your hand.
7. Place 1 generous tablespoon of filling in each and gather up the edges into a small little "purse" and twist/pinch the top to seal the dumpling shut.
8. Steam the dumplings over high heat for 12 minutes. Eat hot and enjoy!

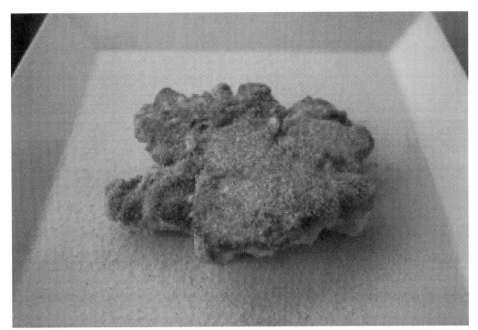

These apple fritters are such a fun, easy recipe that I recommend incorporating in your next Little sleep-over. Similar to pancake dough, this recipe mixes chopped apples and a basic griddled dough to create this autumnal treat.

Easy Apple Fritters

Serves: 12 servings

Ingredients:

- 4 cooking apples (peeled and cored)
- 1 1/4 cups unbleached flour
- 1/2 teaspoon baking powder
- 2 tablespoons sugar
- 2 eggs (separated)
- 1/2 cup milk

Instructions:

1. Peel and cut apples into small chunks
2. Sift together the flour, baking powder and sugar
3. Beat egg yolks and milk together
4. Pour wet ingredients into dry ingredients
5. Fold egg whites into the batter
6. Add apple chunks into the batter and mix evenly
7. Drop tablespoons of batter into hot oil and cook until golden brown on both sides

8. Serve warm with cinnamon sugar on top. Enjoy!

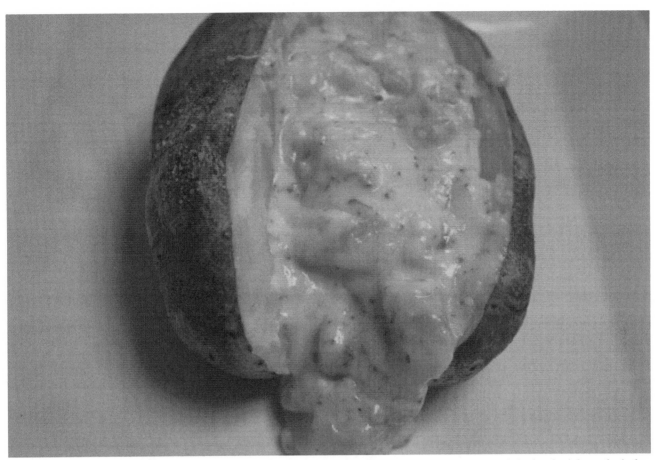

There is a certain fast food chain, which I cannot mention by name who has a red-haired girl as their logo. Their cheesy baked potatoes are good but wait until you try mine.

Cheesy-Broccoli Baked Potato

Serves: 4 servings

Ingredients:

For the Baked Potatoes:

- 4 russet potatoes (2 lb. total)
- 1 Tbsp olive oil
- Salt

For the Broccoli Cheese Sauce:

- ½ lb. frozen broccoli florets
- 3 Tbsp butter
- 3 Tbsp all-purpose flour

- 3 cups whole milk
- ½ tsp salt
- ¼ tsp garlic powder
- 6 oz. medium cheddar, shredded

Instructions:

1. Preheat the oven to 400°F. Take the broccoli out of the freezer and allow it to thaw as the potatoes bake. Once thawed, roughly chop the broccoli into small pieces and then set aside until ready to use.

2. Wash the potatoes well, then dry with paper towel or a clean dish towel. Use a fork to prick several holes in the skin of each potato. Pour the olive oil into a small dish, then use your hands to coat each potato in oil. Place the oil coated potatoes on a baking sheet, and season generously with salt. Bake the potatoes for 45-60 minutes, or until tender all the way through.

3. Towards the end of the baking time, begin to prepare the cheese sauce. Add the butter and flour to a medium saucepan, then place the pot over a medium flame. Whisk the butter and flour together as they melt. Allow the mixture to begin to bubble and foam, whisking continuously. Continue to cook for one minute to remove the raw flour flavor, but do not let the flour begin to brown.

4. Whisk the milk into the butter and flour mixture. Bring the milk up to a simmer, whisking frequently. When it reaches a simmer, it will thicken. Once thick enough to coat a spoon, turn the heat down to the lowest setting. Season the white sauce with the salt and garlic powder.

5. Add a handful of the shredded cheddar to the sauce at a time, whisking until it has fully melted before adding the next handful. Once all of the cheddar has been melted into the sauce, stir in the chopped broccoli. Leave the sauce over a low flame, stirring occasionally, to keep it warm.

6. When the potatoes are finished baking, carefully slice them open. Use a fork to slightly mash the insides of the potatoes. When ready to serve, place each potato on a plate and ladle the broccoli cheese sauce over each potato. Garnish with extra shredded cheddar, if desired.

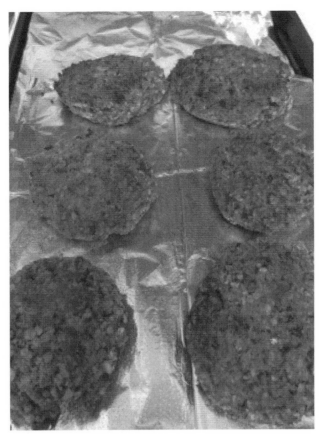

Veggie burger patties are delicious and nutritious without all the fat. Oats bind these patties together while the black beans pack a protein punch.

Veggie Burger Patties

Serves: 6 patties

Ingredients:

- 3 carrots
- 2 bell peppers
- 1 can kidney beans
- 2 green onions
- 1.5 cups quick-cook oats
- A pinch of dried: parsley, oregano, and garlic powder
- A pinch of salt and black pepper

Instructions:

1. Chop up the carrots into a food processor. Then add chopped bell peppers and pulse until minced.

2. Add the chopped green onions, and kidney beans (rinsed) and blend until smooth.
3. Add 1.5 cups quick cook oats and pulse until just combined.
4. Form into patties and pan-sear in a skillet with a drizzle of oil on medium-high heat for 3-4 minutes per side. (Just until it's slightly brown on each side).
5. Then transfer each patty onto a foil-lined baking sheet and bake at 375 degrees (F) for 20 minutes and enjoy!

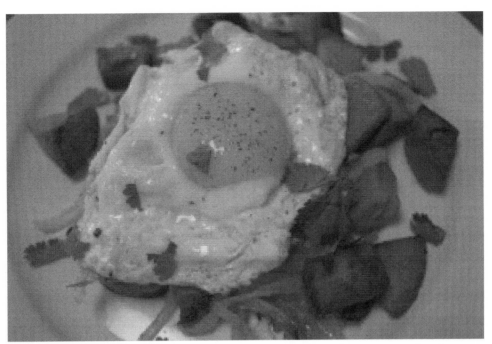

This sweet potato hash is a healthier twist on Saturday morning brunch. Be sure to let the potatoes crisp up in the pan without moving them around much and you're golden.

Sweet Potato Hash and Eggs

Serves: 3 servings

Ingredients:

- 2 yams, peeled and washed
- 1 onion, peeled and sliced
- Cajun seasoning
- Oil for frying

Instructions:

1. Peel, cut and wash your yams. Then cut into cubes. (Don't worry about knife cuts here. Just chop those taters up!)
2. Fill a pot with water and bring to a boil. Put the yams in the boiling water and cook for 10 minutes. (You want them soft enough to be pricked with a fork but not fall apart).
3. Drain the yams and set them into a mixing bowl. Now it's time to season! I used Cajun seasoning because I love to kick things up a notch. But you can alternatively use Old Bay Seasoning, salt, and black pepper, for a savory yet mild flavor. Or you can also use a bit of dried sage and rosemary with salt and pepper, for a more herb-y breakfast potato. Use your palate and get creative!

4. Heat up your oil in a saucepan on high heat. When the oil is hot, test it out with a piece of sweet potato. It should sizzle immediately when you drop it in. If it does, you're ready to fry! Drop in the sweet potatoes and fry for 3 minutes. (This is important: don't touch the potatoes for 3 minutes. Let them brown and sit in the pan!) Then after 3 minutes, flip them over with a spatula. Add your chopped onions. Fry for an additional 3 minutes.

5. Divide into equal portions and top with a fried egg and serve. Enjoy!

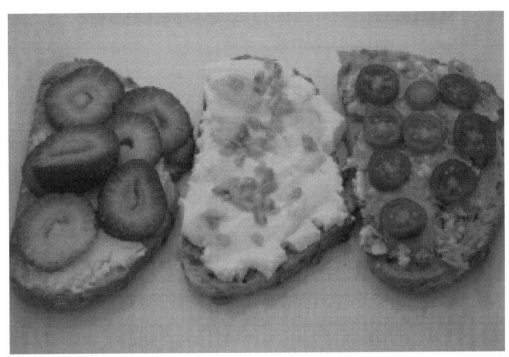

I love getting creative with toast. Use whatever ingredients you have on hand and see what combinations you can come up with. Here are a few of my favorites.

Fancy Toast Party

Serves: 1 serving

Ingredients:

For Strawberry-Cream Cheese-Honey Toast:

- 1 slice sunflower seed bread
- 2 strawberries, sliced
- 2 tbsp. cream cheese
- A drizzle of honey

For Honey-Walnut-Ricotta Toast:

- 1 slice sunflower seed bread
- 2 tbsp. ricotta cheese
- 1 tsp. chopped walnuts
- A drizzle of honey

For Avocado-Feta-Tomato Toast:

- 1 slice sunflower seed bread
- 1 avocado, pitted and mashed
- 3 cherry tomatoes, sliced
- 4 tbsp. feta cheese, mixed into mashed avocado

Instructions:

1. Assemble each toast, serve, and enjoy!

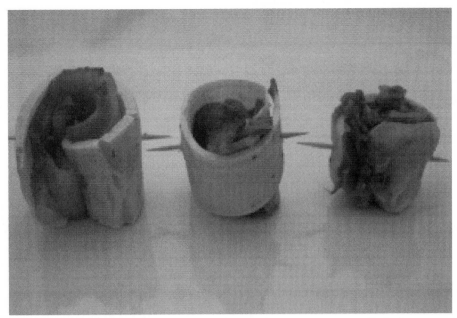

You'll find that the balance of spicy kimchi, savory bacon, and sweet potato really balance each other out in this one-bite appetizer. Surprise your friends when you lay this out at your next party.

Kimchi Sweet Potato Bacon Bites

Serves: 10 bites

Ingredients:

- 2 sweet potatoes, peeled and cut lengthwise through a mandolin
- 10 strips bacon, fried
- 1 cup kimchi, diced

Instructions:

1. Preheat the oven to 400 degrees (F). Begin by running each peeled sweet potato lengthwise through the mandolin so you end up with long, thin strips. Place a piece of parchment paper on a cookie sheet and bake the sweet potatoes in the oven for 6-8 minutes, (checking to see that they don't burn). Remove and let cool.
2. Meanwhile, fry your bacon in a pan until crispy then drain and set aside.
3. Dice up the kimchi into bite sized pieces and set aside.
4. Then it's time to assemble! Grab a ribbon of sweet potato, a piece of bacon, and several pieces of kimchi and place them down on top of each other using the sweet potato as the base. Roll it up and pierce with a toothpick to hold it closed. Serve warm and enjoy!

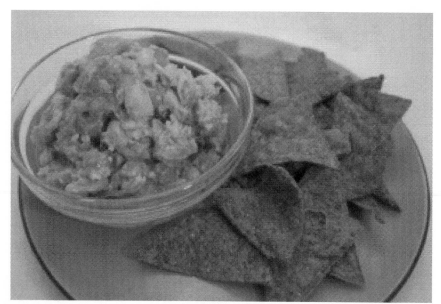

Everybody has their own style and recipe for making guacamole. I prefer mine chunky yet creamy. You can add a few shakes of ground turmeric to up the nutritional value in this easy dip.

Guacamole

Serves: 4 servings (about 1/2 cup per person)

Ingredients:

- 1 tomato, seeded and diced
- 1/2 sweet onion, diced
- 2 avocados, pitted and mashed
- 1 handful coriander/cilantro, diced finely
- 1 lime, juiced
- Salt to taste

Instructions:

1. Grab a mixing bowl and mash up both avocados. Choose how chunky or creamy you like it. (Personally, I mash mine pretty well since we are already adding chopped onion and tomato into the mix).
2. Add your chopped onion, tomato, and cilantro. Mix well.
3. Add the juice of 1 lime and mix well again! Season with salt to taste and serve immediately with some great corn chips! Enjoy!

Chapter IX.

The Power of Music: 100 Songs for Little Space

*F*or as long as humans have been around, we have been making music. Over time, people (mainly those brainy scientists) have discovered that what you listen to matters. Music is a powerful tool that can enhance your Little Space and bring you and your Dom together. Understanding how music can impact you and your D/s relationship is a great place to start. Music has been proven to help soothe and relax people. It can also slow your heart rate and blood pressure. Think about all those times your school teacher played classical music during testing. Does that ring a bell? The music is soothing and therefore allows the mind to gently focus on the task at hand. Music also can be uplifting and promote movement and dance. While in Little Space, many littles may struggle verbally communicating their needs to their Dom. This is especially true when you're having a rotten day. Personally, when I'm having a case of the grumps and I just can't talk about it, my daddy will often use music as a way to get me to "talk" about my feelings. A song can have lyrics that fit how we're feeling, and when we play it, our Dom can better understand what's going on in our mind. Music has the capability to shift and lift our mood after a long day. When you hear "your jam" pop on in your earbuds you can't help but bop your head to the beat. Likewise, sometimes you'll be listening to angry or dark music and notice your mood worsen. You might feel a bit melancholier. Pay attention the next time you're listening to music and tap into your emotions. Ask yourself how you're feeling and see if there is a correlation between what you're listening to, and how you're feeling.

Music can also be an excellent tool to use in long distance D/l relationships. If your relationship is based more in play sessions through the use of Skype or another messenger service, try having a sing-a-long together sometime! I bet you'll have a blast playing music and rocking out together. There are also many apps that encourage users to video stream while singing duets or portions of the song. You can record yourself singing and then send it privately to your friends. This would be such a fun little date to have with your Dom/Domme. Some apps with these features include: Smule, Karaoke-Sing Unlimited Songs, Starmaker- Sing Karaoke, and Red Karaoke Sing & Record. Lastly, there is another platform online called Watch2gether.com which I highly recommend for streaming videos with your Dom/Domme. This site allows users to share a private room (only you as the creator of the room will have the code/link to share with others) to stream videos and watch at the same time. There is a chat box in which you can message as you're watching, and the best part is that it's completely free with no registration required! Watch2gether.com allows users to search for videos from various platforms that it syncs up to including: YouTube, Vimeo, Gfycat, Twitch, Dailymotion, Facebook, Soundcloud, Mixcloud, and W2gSync.

Music can also be a bonding tool for you and your dom/domme. As you grow together in your D/s relationship, share music that reflects your background or culture. It just so happens that my daddy (and husband) is Filipino, while I am Irish-American. As we got to know each other I listened to Filipino music for the first time, and he became immersed in Irish music. Are there songs from your background that you can share with your dominant? Maybe you identify with a regional place and draw music or inspiration from where you live? For example: The Southern U.S. has some incredible Country and Hip-Hop artists, while the Pacific Northwest has birthed some awesome punk rock bands! The U.K. has its own regions and musical influences too. Think about where you live and see if there are bands and songs you can share in your relationship. Finally, everyone has songs that connect with them on a personal level. We all have those songs that make the breath in your throat catch. You hear the song and pause, it's just that powerful. Maybe it evokes a memory, or is a song that your family taught you or maybe it's a religious song that really hits home? Whatever that song is, I encourage you to share it with your Dom/Domme and have that special moment together. They can get to know you on a deeper level simply by sharing that part of yourself.

The final point I wanted to share with you is about using music to deepen your D/l bond. You can incorporate music into play sessions in several different ways. You can bring in musical toys while you're in little space such as: xylophones, recorders, or electronic toys that sing. You can watch shows that are very music and dance oriented including: The Wiggles, Yo Gabba Gabba, and The Electric Company, to name just a few. You can also sing with your Dom/Domme, songs that promote touch. Try incorporating songs that involve hand clapping (ex.: Miss Mary Mac, The Itsy Bitsy Spider, etc.) that allows you and your Dom/Domme to touch hands as you sing together.

I also want to specifically address littles who do incorporate sex into little space. Music can be a powerful tool to use to spark foreplay with your dominant. There are numerous songs to set the mood, and bring fantasies to life. If your dominant likes seeing you dance and sing like the happy little that you are, you can easily put on an upbeat song, a cute onesie, and bring that joy into a more sexual space between the two of you. I truly believe that there is an art to serenading. When you're serenading your dominant try to remember to keep eye contact. The eyes are a window to the soul, and making eye contact with your Dom/Domme shows that you are theirs. Every part of you is tuned into the moment as you sing to them. Lastly, remember that some songs are better than others to have playing while you make love. Think about the beat of the song and the message that you wish to portray as you bring music into the bedroom.

The final point I wish to address with you is finding pleasure in music together as a D/l couple. Music should bring joy, happiness, and enhance your time in little space. Think about attending a free summer concert together. Listening to outdoor music can be a blast and in a casual environment like this, you can pull up a few lawn chairs and discreetly be in little space listening to the music as you rock out together. You and your dom can also play instruments together. This is an excellent activity to stimulate your brain and boost stimulation in the body while making music together. I also recommend that every couple have "their song" that they choose together. D/l couples are no exception. Find a song with your dom that resonates with you both. Make it a bonding activity and then create a whole playlist together! It's something you can turn to and use for many fun times.

Now without further ado, here are 100 songs all available on YouTube to spark inspiration for your own Little playlist:

1. **A La Nanita Nana** By: The Cheetah Girls
2. **Perfect Day** By: Miriam Stockley
3. **Song of the Sea** By: Nolwenn Leroy
4. **We Are One** By: Lion King 2 Soundtrack
5. **Crazy For This Girl** By: Evan and Jaron
6. **Beautiful Soul** By: Jesse McCartney
7. **Never Had a Dream Come True** By: S Club 7
8. **Bubbly** By: Colbie Calliat
9. **Banana Pancakes** By: Jack Johnson
10. **Better Together** By: Jack Johnson
11. **What a Wonderful World** By: Louis Armstrong
12. **When You Wish Upon a Star** By: Cliff Edwards
13. **Lava** By: Disney
14. **Return to Pooh Corner** By: Kenny Loggins
15. **My Favorite Things** By: Julie Andrews
16. **Feed the Birds** By: Julie Andrews
17. **All the Pretty Little Ponies** By: Kenny Loggins
18. **Pure Imagination, Somewhere Out There, Neverland Medley** By: Kenny Loggins
19. **Rainbow Connection** By: Kermit the Frog
20. **Somewhere Over the Rainbow** By: Israel Kamakawiwo'ole
21. **Play That Song** By: Train
22. **Rhythm of Love** By: Plain White T's
23. **Girls Chase Boys** By: Ingrid Michaelson
24. **Best Day of My Life** By: American Authors
25. **Good Time** By: Owl City ft. Carly Rae Jepsen
26. **Cheerleader** By: OMI
27. **What Makes You Different** By: The Backstreet Boys
28. **Like Me** By: Teen Beach Movie Soundtrack
29. **I Want To Hold Your Hand** By: The Beatles
30. **Just Like Romeo and Juliet** By: The Reflections
31. **A Summer Song** By: Chad and Jeremy
32. **Say Hey (I Love You)** By: Michael Franti and Spearhead
33. **Another Day in Paradise** By: Phil Collins
34. **Good Life** By: Onerepublic
35. **Dance With Me Tonight** By: Olly Murs
36. **Upside Down** By: Jack Johnson
37. **Tinker Bell** By: April
38. **Beep Beep** By: SNSD
39. **Sleepsong** By: Secret Garden Soundtrack
40. **Fairy Nightsongs** By: Gary Stadler

41. **Offshore Wind** By: The Pirateers
42. **Davy Jones** By: Fialeja
43. **Daughter of the Moon** By: Adriana Figueroa
44. **Brahm's Lullaby** By: Jewel
45. **Wolfsong** By: Denny Schneidemesser
46. **Never Smile at a Crocodile** By: Peter Pan Soundtrack
47. **When Will My Life Begin** By: Tangled Soundtrack
48. **California Gurls** By: Katy Perry ft. Snoop Dogg
49. **There She Goes** By: The La's
50. **American Girl** By: Bonnie McKee
51. **Sakura** By: Ikimono Gakari
52. **MitchiriNecko March Song**
53. **You Are My Senpai Song**
54. **Happy** By: Pharrell Williams
55. **Wake Me Up Before You Go-Go** By: Wham!
56. **Walking On Sunshine** By: Katrina and the Waves
57. **Brave** By: Sara Bareilles
58. **The Lazy Song** By: Bruno Mars
59. **Shut Up and Dance** By: Walk the Moon
60. **Firework** By: Katy Perry
61. **Hey, Soul Sister** By: Train
62. **MMMBop** By: Hanson
63. **I Feel Good** By: James Brown
64. **You Get What You Give** By: New Radicals
65. **Dancing Queen** By: ABBA
66. **Girls Just Want to Have Fun** By: Cyndi Lauper
67. **Better When I'm Dancin** By: Meghan Trainor
68. **Vanilla Twilight** By: Owl City
69. **Wannabe** By: Spice Girls
70. **Butterfly Kisses** By: Bob Dylan
71. **You Can Be King Again** By: Lauren Aquilina
72. **I Won't Give Up** By: Jason Mraz
73. **I'm Yours** By: Jason Mraz
74. **Island in the Sun** By: Weezer
75. **Buddy Holly** By: Weezer
76. **Accidentally In Love** By: Counting Crows
77. **The Way You Love Me** By: Faith Hill
78. **This Kiss** By: Faith Hill
79. **Summer Sunshine** By: The Corrs
80. **Angel** By: The Corrs
81. **Uptown Girl** By: Westlife

82. **That's the Way It Is** By: Celine Dion
83. **Invisible** By: Clay Aiken
84. **Bumble Bee** By: Bambee
85. **Boom Boom Boom Boom** By: Venga Boys
86. **Go Go Go Go** By: 89ers (Ti-Mo Remix)
87. **Stamp On the Ground** By: Italobrothers
88. **Waka Waka** By: Shakira
89. **Whenever, Wherever** By: Shakira
90. **Barbie Girl** By: Aqua
91. **PonPonPon** By: Kyary Pamyu Pamyu
92. **Party** By: Girls' Generation
93. **Our Last Summer** By: Mamma Mia Soundtrack
94. **Lay All Your Love On Me** By: Mamma Mia Soundtrack
95. **Music of the Night** By: Andrew Lloyd Webber
96. **Touch the Sky** By: Brave Soundtrack
97. **He Mele No Lilo** By: Lilo & Stitch Soundtrack
98. **Hawaiian Roller Coaster Ride** By: Lilo & Stitch Soundtrack
99. **Lavender's Blue Dilly Dilly** By: Cinderella Soundtrack (2015)
100. **A Dream is a Wish Your Heart Makes** By: Cinderella Soundtrack

Chapter X:

Time Out and Other Forms of Punishment For Your Little

*I*n order to understand how you should punish your Little, perhaps we should begin at why you implement punishment at all. Punishment is a delicate subject within the D/s world and more so within the D/l community because the very nature of littles is far more sensitive than other paths of submission. So, what is the purpose of punishment and why is it so important? Let's think of punishment as a form of love between the dominant and their little. Just as parents use punishment to guide and correct behavior deemed inappropriate, so too does the dom use punishment to guide their submissive into appropriate action. Introducing the topic of punishment is usually given during the training period at the start of any D/s relationship. The dominant will address rules that they have for their submissive. They will then clearly state (sometimes even within the D/s contract) what form of punishment they wish to use should a rule be broken.

There are clear Do's and Don'ts when it comes to implementing punishment that every dominant should adhere to. Here are several rules to keep in mind:

- **Do** consult with the submissive as to what punishment type you (the dominant) wish to use. There may be past trauma and limitations that a form of punishment can trigger. The aim of punishing a little is to gently correct behavior, not scar the individual. Change your form of punishment to work with the little and their needs.
- **Do** be mindful of the language you use during giving out a punishment. Strong, verbal commands (while important) can easily overwhelm a little. A wise dominant is one who can discipline their little without having to shout. Emotional abuse is never acceptable for any reason.
- **Do** encourage your little to adhere to your rules through external reward. Again, the aim is to praise and encourage good behavior, and gently correct bad behavior. Give your little a reason to adhere to the rules with little treats, snacks, etc.
- **Don't** use punishment as a means to further dominate your submissive. If you want a masochist, then look for that type of submissive. Littles are submissives who need lots of attention, care, and snuggles. They generally don't respond well to strict, corporal punishment.
- **Don't** use punishment to leave permanent marks on your Little's skin. The body of a Little is one to be cherished. Never aim to mark, brand, tattoo, or scar your Little. If hardcore masochism is a part of your play, then consent from the submissive before any action is taken should be adhered to above all else.
- Lastly, **NEVER**, ever threaten to take away the relationship or ignore your Little as a form of punishment. The little places their trust, love, and care into your hands as the dominant. You hold their fragile, emotional well-being in the palm of your hand. This is a huge responsibility not to be taken lightly. If you threaten to end the relationship, you shatter all trust within the D/l bond.

Another aspect of punishment that dominants must be aware of is the Little's pain threshold. Every Little is different in the level of pain they can endure and what tools of punishment they are comfortable with. Always have safe words established so that you, the dominant, can be aware when your submissive needs the punishment to end immediately. Also, you the submissive, need to place comfort within the use of safe words and know that when you say. For example, "Yellow" may mean "slow down- now! I need a moment to regroup", and your dominant will do so immediately. Having safe words shows respect and trust within the relationship. All D/s relationships should have safe words established during the time of making a contract. If for any reason either party does not wish to have safe words, I encourage you to walk away. This is a major "red flag" and can lead to dangerous situations.

As the dominant, you also need to decide what tools of punishment to use on your little. Should you use a crop? How about your hand, while the little is bent over the knee? Maybe you want to use a hairbrush to paddle their behind? Deciding what tools to use is an important decision and one to think about carefully. Littles are adults who have a need to regress within the safety, and privacy of little space, with you as the dominant, guiding and protecting them. Yes, they can handle spankings that make their rump red or pink. But do littles want to be gagged, flogged, and tied up to a rack? Unless that is a topic that comes up during the point of establishing your contract together, then I would advise you to stay away from deep forms of bondage with your little.

Punishing your little should be something that keeps the submissive within the mindset of little space. Generally, spanking over the knee is advised as the primary physical form of punishment. There is a stark difference between a Master's punishments, and a Daddy or Mommy's punishments, that all submissive should be aware of. A Master is a dominant who is generally stricter towards their submissive. When a submissive enters into a relationship with their Dom/Domme, they understand that the punishment will be swift and more physical in nature because the other paths of submission (slave, masochists, domestic servants, pony girls, pain pigs, kajira, etc.) all require surrendering total submission to the dominant. The power exchange between both consenting adults grants the dominant the ability to use punishment in a more physical manner. Littles aren't like the other submissive paths.

Littles are submissives who have fluid, yet deep power exchange with their dominant. They are fiercely loyal, gentle, bubbly, and deeply loving towards their dominant. In return, dominants gain a happy, optimistic, ray of sunshine in their life from their Little. Unlike Master's who can be more independent between play sessions, dominants of a Little usually must keep a close pulse on their submissive at all times. This is because the little is a deeply feeling person who yearns to regress many times a day. Punishment from a daddy or mommy is something that must be gentler. The Master leaves marks on their submissive to reprimand and change behavior; the Daddy or Mommy leaves marks on the littles mind to change behavior. "Go to the corner and think about what you did wrong" is a common phrase said in the D/l community. The Daddy/Mommy knows their little so intimately that they needn't use physical tools to get their littles attention. The little will feel deep remorse for their infraction when they see their dom's eyes fill with shame and disappointment in them. The little strives to keep their dom happy, so there are ways to punish your little without laying a finger on them at all.

One way to achieve punishment without physical spankings is to incorporate a time out mat. Amazon sells portable time out mats for around $13 USD that is a cloth mat with a bullseye in the center that reads "Time Out". So, your little will understand immediately where they need to sit, as you tell them why they are being punished. The psychological aspect of sitting in time out to reflect is an obstacle for most littles. Having to be quiet and think about their actions can have a far greater impact than any spanking would. Other dominants place a traditional time out chair in the corner of the room and make their little sit in it facing the wall as punishment. Lastly, another form of non-physical punishment that can be used with a Little is withholding orgasm. There are many online retailers that sell chastity belts for women in which the dominant can place on their little and hold the key so that their submissive is unable to masturbate or achieve orgasm until the punishment is over. This can be quite the struggle (and punishment!) for a little with a high libido yet, it can be deeply effective in gently guiding and correcting their behavior.

It's no secret that littles have a reputation of "bratting" their Dom/Domme. Go online and search "DDLG clothing" and you're likely to find clothing which reads: crybaby, brat, whiner, etc. There is a misconception that littles like to brat their Dom/Domme and that many do so. To understand the issue of bratting (which ultimately leads the dominant to have to punish the Little) it is vital to understand why littles brat to begin with. Littles brat their dominant for attention. Whether the attention is negative or positive is irrelevant. They want attention from their Dom/Domme, and they want it now! So, they do things, and break rules, to achieve the immediate goal of getting it. The wise Dom/Domme would see this and know that behavior like that is unacceptable and needs immediate correction. However, there is a deeper issue with bratting that needs to be addressed.

When you enter into a D/s relationship it is born from a place of respect, trust, love, and obedience. This is the same with a D/l relationship too. The little must go through the period of training with their dominant to establish trust and respect, as well as to understand what the dom expects from them as their submissive. When a little brats, one must ask if the submissive has been properly trained. Yes, every little acts out every now and then, life happens. But if a little is bratting often, then there are several issues at hand. One, is that they are showing a lack of respect and obedience to their dom/domme which goes against the very nature of D/s relationships. Secondly, bratting often calls into question if the submissive is too immature to handle an adult, consensual relationship like a D/s relationship. If they are acting out often, are they fit to be a sub? And lastly, dominants (especially Daddies and Mommies), are only human. Yes, they are incredibly kind, loving, and patient people. But making a dom/domme deal with bratting regularly is undue stress that just isn't fair to place upon them. This is something dominants should keep in mind while establishing a bond with their submissive.

So, if bratting frequently is unhealthy to a relationship, then what should a dominant do when their submissive does act out? What do you do when your little can't get into little space? Or what if they have their period and feel miserable? What should the dom/domme do when their little is having a horrible day? The answer is quite simple. Use these situations to "shine" and gain deeper trust, love, and respect from your little one by being there for them as the best caregiver you can be. If you little is having trouble slipping into little space, try letting them vent to you as "big me". Let them get it all off of their chest as you hold them close. Then see if they feel like snuggling up with a snack and a movie. Gently guide them into a place of comfort and emotional care as they ease into little space. If your little is on their monthly cycle, ask them if there is a special food you can pick up for them. (Odds are, it's chocolate!). Snuggle up close to them, and just be there with love, food, and a heating pad. Your little will remember that in a couple of days after the pain is gone, that you were there. They will trust and love you so much more deeply because you were there when they felt awful. You demonstrated your ability to be a caregiver when they needed you most and that is what counts! In return, you will find your submissive being far more obedient and the bond that you two have will deepen, grow, and flourish. And really, that is what it's all about.

Chapter XI:

How to Thrive Being a Solo Little

*T*he journey of self-discovery is a beautiful one when discovering you're a Little. You have questions and you begin to research the answers. You get to tap into parts of yourself that have yet to be discovered and unearth old pleasures that you felt during childhood. It's a beautiful time of self-reflection, but often times Littles believe that they need a dominant to actually be a Little. This couldn't be farther from the truth! Honey, you are a Little whether or not a Dom/Domme comes knocking on your door to sweep you off of your feet. Being Little is a who you are, not who you're with! In this chapter I want to focus on how you can thrive as a solo Little.

My fellow Little, it all starts from within. You, (yes, YOU) are truly beautiful. There is no one else in the world just like you. Trust me when I say that the beginning of your journey into being a Little is getting to know yourself better. In this time and space as a solo Little you have the opportunity to explore who you are as a person, what things you like (And don't), what type of little you see yourself as, and what type of Dom/Domme you need. I implore you to dig deep and discover these parts of yourself because when you do meet a dominant, they will be asking you all of these questions and hoping that you have the answers. Are you ready to get to know yourself better? Yes? Then let's go!

Who are you? Only you can answer that. But if someone were to ask you, "describe yourself to me", what would you say? Would you immediately gravitate towards your physical attributes? Or would you talk about who you are on the inside? Sexual attraction is an important part of traditional D/s relationships, but it's who you are as a person that is going to sustain the connection with your Dom/Domme. So how would you describe yourself? Are you shy or outgoing? What are some things you enjoy doing for fun? What is a fear of yours? Allow your mind to wander as you ponder these questions. Dig deep within yourself and think about who you are, and if there are parts of yourself that you want to nurture and change. As you meet and connect with a dominant, they will help guide you with tasks and goals for you to work on these parts that you wish to change. But before they can help you, you need to be able to articulate with your dom what things you want to change about yourself!

There are many kinks and fetishes out there for you to explore. As a solo little, another aspect you should investigate are kinks that interest you. Don't worry, you don't need to go running off to the nearest adult shop to buy a bunch of toys (though you can...). Instead, go online and search "list of kinks, fetishes, and tropes" and read about various ones. There are literally hundreds of kinks out there. You can be a little, but also have another kink that interests you. This is completely, and totally normal. You might be wondering, "yes, but why would I want to do that if I'm a solo Little??". Your dominant will also be asking you what turns you on, what fantasies do you have, and are there any kinks that you've tried or wish to try. He/She will guide you gently into exploring these parts of yourself. It's what a dominant does. For example: there are many submissives who engage in pet play. Along with being a Little, they gather accessories (pet ear headbands, a tail, etc.) to wear in play sessions and assume the role of their dominant's pet. Their dom/domme guides them into exploring this kink and allows them to dive deeply into this fantasy. (If you are interested in pet play, there are many books available to further discuss this kink, as well as groups such as thechateau.org, that host in-person meet-ups for pet play).

Another aspect of being a solo little is preparing yourself to be a submissive to a dominant. You don't need to have a dominant to be a submissive, but if having a dom/domme is something you wish to have in the future then you need to have yourself as established and prepared both physically and mentally for all that it entails. I have created a 25-day training schedule for the solo Little to give you general tasks and a guideline as you grow more comfortable with yourself. This guide focuses on the following:

- Following a healthy and manageable morning routine
- Finding your own fashion style while still feeling little
- Carving out time for 15 minutes of meditation per day
- Find snacks that keep that little spark within while you are out and about
- Taking time for daily reflection questions in a journal at night
- Watch D/s themed movies (and complete the activity below associated with each movie) to get you thinking about what to look for in a dominant
- Exercise for 20 minutes per day at your mobility level and keep those muscles healthy
- Establish a nighttime routine
- And get plenty of quality rest at night. A rested little is a happy little!

Are you ready to begin your training as a Little? Then let's jump in together!!

The 25-Day Training Plan for Littles

Day 1: Self-Acceptance

Hello, Little One! Congratulations on the start of your Little training. Over the next 25 days you will be completing tasks and activities to prepare you for connecting with a dominant. The goal of this training is to help ground and center you. The more you understand yourself and what you seek in a dominant, the more successful you will be in your future relationship. It all starts from within.

That said, let's begin your training right now. Today's focus is going to be on self-acceptance. In order to get where you're going, you must first accept where you are right here and now. As you dive into the world of DDLG/LB you will be filled with images on social media of Littles in all shapes and sizes. It's easy to envy those who have a different figure then you. But the goal of today's exercise is to learn to accept all parts of yourself just as you are. You don't need to fit into a specific onesie size. There is no "bar" or standard that Littles should meet in how patient they are, or if they act a certain way. Who your "Little Me" is inside, is specific and unique to you. You don't need to be anyone other than you. Now I want you to close your eyes and think about who you are. What are your talents? What are things that you know you excel in? Look at yourself in a mirror. Go on.... look! This is who you are right here, right now. Your curves are all you and it's truly beautiful. I want you to say to yourself, **"I accept who I am today"** out loud.

You might not believe that at first, but a Little who is confident in themselves is someone that can relay to a dominant what they need, so we will keep working on your confidence and self-acceptance. Wrap your arms around yourself and give yourself a giant hug! It may feel silly but let's pause for a moment. Your body has been growing and sustaining you for a long, long time! How miraculous is that?! In all of the junk food you've eaten and the many miles you've walked throughout life, your body has been with you every literal step of the way. Give yourself a hug and let's pause in a moment of gratitude that your body has led you to the present where you can be aware of who you are and how you are. You've made it and that is something to rejoice!

Today you will begin your daily routine that includes self-care. While this popular term is thrown around quite a bit, the importance behind it is significant. Caring for yourself is an act of love and self-acceptance. Every time you brush your teeth, or wash your face, you are choosing to put your needs as a priority. And you should, because you're worth it! Focus on completing your tasks today around the daily schedule you already have. Living a Little lifestyle means weaving together Big Me and Little Me. It will take some time to put the two together seamlessly, but over the course of the training and beyond. I know you will find your own rhythm. Enjoy this journey with yourself, my fellow Little, this is a special time for you to fall in love with yourself and nourish yourself, body, mind, and soul.

Day 1 Tasks:

Task #1: Complete Your Morning Routine
- Drink 1 glass of water as soon as you wake up

- Wash your face
- Brush your teeth
- Throw your shower towel into the dryer (if available) and have it tumbling on low-medium heat while you hop into the shower.
- Shower up. While in the shower, think of a song you used to love as a child. Sing that song to yourself as you lather up. Then wrap yourself up in your warm towel afterward. Ahhh...
- Take time to pick out an outfit that is both comfortable, yet makes you feel pretty.
- Put on sunscreen and Chapstick
- Lotion your skin with baby lotion

Task #2: Meditate for 15 minutes

If you have a phone, I want you to download the FREE app. Headspace. It has guided meditation apps that are picked by the program based upon your current mood. If you do not have a phone, go onto YouTube and follow a 15-minute guided meditation video. Allow your breathing to calm and relax your body. Let go of your stresses and fears. Simply be. This daily practice is designed to train you to build up patience in sitting still as you will need to do for your dominant in the future.

Task #3: Browse DDLG/LB Fashion Online

Begin browsing fashion online to formulate your own unique little style! You can also see previous chapters (III., IV., and V. in this book for product and clothing suggestions). There is a style for everyone. Go and find yours!

Task #4: Time to start your normal day, but don't forget your Little snacks!

Whether you're going to school, or staying at home, as you're doing your normal daily schedule I want you to take several breaks throughout the day to refuel with a glass of water and a small snack. These snacks should specifically remind you of Little Me. Some suggestions include: goldfish crackers, animal crackers, cheese cubes, lunchables, cheerios, etc.

Task #5: Stretch those muscles for 20 minutes of exercise!

This act of self-care will keep you feeling good and your body strong. Pick an activity that you already enjoy doing and exercise for 20 minutes.

Task #6: Evening D/s Movie

Every day for the next 25 days I want you to watch a movie that I've hand-picked that is designed to make you think about qualities that dominants should have. Characters in these movies all portray traits that most dom's exude. Think about the relationship dynamics and then follow up in Task #6 with your evening journal reflection letter.

Tonight's D/s Movie is: *A Cinderella Story (2004)*

Task #7: Evening Journal Reflection

Now that your day is starting to wind down and you have completed your first D/s movie, I want you to do an evening journal reflection. Instead of a typical diary entry, I want you to write a letter to your future dominant. You can begin by saying: Dear Future Dom... or Dear Dominant... or Dear Daddy/Mommy.... write what feels natural to you. Think about the qualities you want your dominant to have. Write about wishes you hope for, and dates you want to do with them. Write about the movie you watched tonight and things that are going on in your life. This journal will be a special gift to give your dom when you finally come together.

Task #8: Complete Your Night Time Routine
- Drink 1 glass of water
- Brush your teeth
- Turn off all social media and computers. Power down for the night.
- Pull on fresh pajamas
- If you have a picture book, (or checked one out from the library), lay down in bed and quietly read your book. If you don't have a picture book, listen to a read aloud picture book on YouTube. (There are bunches of videos!)
- Reduce your room lighting to a simple side lamp or fairy lights. Quiet the mind.
- Turn on soft lullaby music or classical music on YouTube
- As you begin to feel groggy, turn everything off, snuggle up to your plushie and drift off to sleep. (Make sure to get those 7-8 hours of rest in!).

Day 2: Easing Into Little Space

Welcome to Day 2 of your Little Training! Today we will focus on easing into little space. Little space is a state of mind. It is the suspension of your daily life, routine, the way you feel about your adult body, etc. and instead embracing your inner child. Once upon a time you were a child and the world looked very different. You might have had a vivid imagination. Your favorite toys come to life in your mind's eye as you created pretend play scenarios. In this training, I want to unearth those feelings that lay dormant in your mind and bring them to the surface again. We will start by using a single object to transition into little space.

I want you to find an object from your childhood that reminds you of a good memory. This can be an old plushie or another toy. It can be a picture of you as a child. Maybe it's a holiday ornament that holds significant meaning. Each Little has their own favorite items, and now it is time to establish yours. Do you have your item in hand? Good. This will be your anchor for little space. Close your eyes and envision what you were like as a child. Feel that sense of lightness. You have the ability to be happy. All of those adult responsibilities don't exist in Little space. Your only job is to be happy, carefree, laugh, and feel joy in the world. The world is your oyster now because you are a child. You are Little You.

I welcome you to sit somewhere comfortably and remain in this space of little me. If you have privacy and feel comfortable doing so, open your eyes and try playing with your toy. Do what feels natural as you remain in that headspace. If you don't have privacy, then remain in quiet meditation within little space. Your "Little Me" is a state of mind, not a physical place. It is who you are, so you can keep it with you like a beautiful secret at all times. Let your mind wander as you dance and dream about all of the wonderful things in the world. You can daydream of rainbows, glitter, your favorite songs, anything really! Allow your mind to feel happy and at peace. This is the joy of going into little space.

When you're ready, slowly ease back into "Big Me" space. Open your eyes or gently lay down your toy. Reflect on how you feel. Take a moment and sit in stillness as you bask in the effects of this exercise. Then, when you're ready to proceed, go ahead and begin your daily tasks.

Day 2 Tasks:

Task #1: Complete Your Morning Routine
- Drink 1 glass of water as soon as you wake up
- Wash your face
- Brush your teeth
- Throw your shower towel into the dryer (if available) and have it tumbling on low-medium heat while you hop into the shower.
- Shower up. While in the shower, think of a song you used to love as a child. Sing that song to yourself as you lather up. Then wrap yourself up in your warm towel afterward. Ahhh...

- Take time to pick out an outfit that is both comfortable, yet makes you feel pretty.
- Put on sunscreen and Chapstick
- Lotion your skin with baby lotion

Task #2: Meditate for 15 minutes

If you have a phone, I want you to download the FREE app. Headspace. It has guided meditation apps that are picked by the program based upon your current mood. If you do not have a phone, go onto YouTube and follow a 15-minute guided meditation video. Allow your breathing to calm and relax your body. Let go of your stresses and fears. Simply be. This daily practice is designed to train you to build up patience in sitting still as you will need to do for your dominant in the future.

Task #3: Browse DDLG/LB Fashion Online

Begin browsing fashion online to formulate your own unique little style! You can also see previous chapters (III., IV., and V. in this book for product and clothing suggestions). There is a style for everyone. Go and find yours!

Task #4: Time to start your normal day, but don't forget your Little snacks!

Whether you're going to school, or staying at home, as you're doing your normal daily schedule I want you to take several breaks throughout the day to refuel with a glass of water and a small snack. These snacks should specifically remind you of Little Me. Some suggestions include: goldfish crackers, animal crackers, cheese cubes, lunchables, cheerios, etc.

Task #5: Stretch those muscles for 20 minutes of exercise!

This act of self-care will keep you feeling good and your body strong. Pick an activity that you already enjoy doing and exercise for 20 minutes.

Task #6: Evening D/s Movie

Every day for the next 25 days I want you to watch a movie that I've hand-picked that is designed to make you think about qualities that dominants should have. Characters in these movies all portray traits that most dom's exude. Think about the relationship dynamics and then follow up in Task #6 with your evening journal reflection letter.

Tonight's D/s Movie is: *The Duff (2015)*

Task #7: Evening Journal Reflection

Now that your day is starting to wind down and you have completed your first D/s movie, I want you to do an evening journal reflection. Instead of a typical diary entry, I want you to write a letter to your future dominant. You can begin by saying: Dear Future Dom... or Dear Dominant... or Dear Daddy/Mommy.... write what feels natural to you. Think about the qualities you want your dominant to have. Write about wishes you hope for, and dates you want to do with them. Write about the movie you watched tonight and things that are going on in your life. This journal will be a special gift to give your dom when you finally come together.

Task #8: Complete Your Night Time Routine

- Drink 1 glass of water
- Brush your teeth
- Turn off all social media and computers. Power down for the night.
- Pull on fresh pajamas
- If you have a picture book, (or checked one out from the library), lay down in bed and quietly read your book. If you don't have a picture book, listen to a read aloud picture book on YouTube. (There are bunches of videos!)
- Reduce your room lighting to a simple side lamp or fairy lights. Quiet the mind.
- Turn on soft lullaby music or classical music on YouTube
- As you begin to feel groggy, turn everything off, snuggle up to your plushie and drift off to sleep. (Make sure to get those 7-8 hours of rest in!).

Day 3: Entering Little Space with the Mind Alone

Welcome to Day 3 of your Little Training! Today will focus on getting into Little space using nothing more than your mind. Many people think that in order to be a Little you must wear a onesie, or be surrounded by toys, or have a full-blown nursery! The truth is that there will be many times where you are unable to enter a play session entirely. You will yearn to go into little space, but life just gets in the way. That is when you retreat into a mental Little space. For this exercise, I encourage you to find a quiet, comfortable spot where you can be alone for a few minutes. Once you're ready to relax and unwind, then begin this exercise.

Begin by sitting in a comfortable position and closing your eyes. Envision yourself in your favorite little outfit. Even if you don't own it, envision yourself in a little outfit that you've seen online or perhaps in a magazine. Allow your mind to daydream and wander. Enter that headspace of feeling Little. Suspend any doubts or other thoughts. If a thought does come along, acknowledge it, and like releasing a petal into a breeze, let the thought drift away. Focus on remaining in little space. What are you doing right now in your mind? Are you playing with blocks and building a tower? Are you playing with dolls? Maybe you're outside running through the grass in bare feet! Feel that space completely. Allow your other senses to suspend and enter little space. Feel the wooden blocks against your fingertips with their rough edges. Feel the warm grass beneath your feet and the way the warmth of the sun hits your face. Relax and dream...

When you're ready to return to the present, open your eyes. How are you feeling? What emotions are bubbling up? Acknowledge these feelings. It's okay to let the emotion flow through you. Little space is a place of safety and love. You are safe and who you are entirely is welcomed and embraced. After you've taken some time for reflection, please move on to complete your Day 3 tasks.

Day 3 Tasks:

Task #1: Complete Your Morning Routine
- Drink 1 glass of water as soon as you wake up
- Wash your face
- Brush your teeth
- Throw your shower towel into the dryer (if available) and have it tumbling on low-medium heat while you hop into the shower.
- Shower up. While in the shower, think of a song you used to love as a child. Sing that song to yourself as you lather up. Then wrap yourself up in your warm towel afterward. Ahhh...
- Take time to pick out an outfit that is both comfortable, yet makes you feel pretty.
- Put on sunscreen and Chapstick
- Lotion your skin with baby lotion

Task #2: Meditate for 15 minutes

If you have a phone, I want you to download the FREE app. Headspace. It has guided meditation apps that are picked by the program based upon your current mood. If you do not have a phone, go onto YouTube and follow a 15-minute guided meditation video. Allow your breathing to calm and relax your body. Let go of your stresses and fears. Simply be. This daily practice is designed to train you to build up patience in sitting still as you will need to do for your dominant in the future.

Task #3: Browse DDLG/LB Fashion Online

Begin browsing fashion online to formulate your own unique little style! You can also see previous chapters (III., IV., and V. in this book for product and clothing suggestions). There is a style for everyone. Go and find yours!

Task #4: Time to start your normal day, but don't forget your Little snacks!

Whether you're going to school, or staying at home, as you're doing your normal daily schedule I want you to take several breaks throughout the day to refuel with a glass of water and a small snack. These snacks should specifically remind you of Little Me. Some suggestions include: goldfish crackers, animal crackers, cheese cubes, lunchables, cheerios, etc.

Task #5: Stretch those muscles for 20 minutes of exercise!

This act of self-care will keep you feeling good and your body strong. Pick an activity that you already enjoy doing and exercise for 20 minutes.

Task #6: Evening D/s Movie

Every day for the next 25 days I want you to watch a movie that I've hand-picked that is designed to make you think about qualities that dominants should have. Characters in these movies all portray traits that most dom's exude. Think about the relationship dynamics and then follow up in Task #6 with your evening journal reflection letter.

Tonight's D/s Movie is: *She's All That (1999)*

Task #7: Evening Journal Reflection

Now that your day is starting to wind down and you have completed your first D/s movie, I want you to do an evening journal reflection. Instead of a typical diary entry, I want you to write a letter to your future dominant. You can begin by saying: Dear Future Dom... or Dear Dominant... or Dear Daddy/Mommy.... write what feels natural to you. Think about the qualities you want your dominant to have. Write about wishes you hope for, and dates you want to do with them. Write about the movie you watched tonight and things that are going on in your life. This journal will be a special gift to give your dom when you finally come together.

Task #8: Complete Your Night Time Routine
- Drink 1 glass of water
- Brush your teeth

- Turn off all social media and computers. Power down for the night.
- Pull on fresh pajamas
- If you have a picture book, (or checked one out from the library), lay down in bed and quietly read your book. If you don't have a picture book, listen to a read aloud picture book on YouTube. (There are bunches of videos!)
- Reduce your room lighting to a simple side lamp or fairy lights. Quiet the mind.
- Turn on soft lullaby music or classical music on YouTube
- As you begin to feel groggy, turn everything off, snuggle up to your plushie and drift off to sleep. (Make sure to get those 7-8 hours of rest in!).

Day 4: What Little Path Attracts You?

Welcome to Day 4 of your Little training! In Chapters III., IV., and V. we discussed various types of Littles within the community. To review, there are: adult babies (AB), Littles, and Middles. However, some Littles also blend other kinks and fetishes into their Little space (such as pet play, role play scenes, bondage, etc.). For now, let's stick with these three main groups. Today I want you to think about all three groups and reflect if there is one path that naturally attracts you. Are you curious about being an adult baby? Does the thought of slipping on a onesie and being snuggled by a dominant as they bottle feed you, excite you? Do you yearn to be a Little and dance like a little ray of sunshine as you play with your toys? Are you eager to try on a school uniform and be playful yet flirty as you experiment with being a Middle? Sit back and reflect on which group of the D/l community resonates with you.

You may not know which path attracts you yet, and that is perfectly fine too! The point of this exercise is to get your brain thinking about which path you'd like to try out first. You might try one aspect of being a Little and find that it doesn't click with you at all. Don't give up! Try something else until you find an activity that resonates with who you are. Yesterday you meditated into Little space with nothing more than your mind. Reflect on what you were thinking about. Were you an elementary-aged child? Were you an infant or toddler? Or were you a teenager? Whatever age you regressed to in your mind is a good indication of where to begin your journey into the Little community. You can refer back to the chapters on each Little path to read about characteristics and qualities that each type of Little has. There are also product and store suggestions for you to look at online to begin to get a feel of what items other littles use. I cannot stress enough for you to find clothing, products, etc. that work specifically for you!

Now that you have an idea of where to start investigating, go ahead and take time to explore that path of the Little community. Then when you're ready, focus on your day 4 tasks.

Day 4 Tasks:

Task #1: Complete Your Morning Routine
- Drink 1 glass of water as soon as you wake up
- Wash your face
- Brush your teeth
- Throw your shower towel into the dryer (if available) and have it tumbling on low-medium heat while you hop into the shower.
- Shower up. While in the shower, think of a song you used to love as a child. Sing that song to yourself as you lather up. Then wrap yourself up in your warm towel afterward. Ahhh...
- Take time to pick out an outfit that is both comfortable, yet makes you feel pretty.
- Put on sunscreen and Chapstick
- Lotion your skin with baby lotion

Task #2: Meditate for 15 minutes

If you have a phone, I want you to download the FREE app. Headspace. It has guided meditation apps that are picked by the program based upon your current mood. If you do not have a phone, go onto YouTube and follow a 15-minute guided meditation video. Allow your breathing to calm and relax your body. Let go of your stresses and fears. Simply be. This daily practice is designed to train you to build up patience in sitting still as you will need to do for your dominant in the future.

Task #3: Browse DDLG/LB Fashion Online

Begin browsing fashion online to formulate your own unique little style! You can also see previous chapters (III., IV., and V. in this book for product and clothing suggestions). There is a style for everyone. Go and find yours!

Task #4: Time to start your normal day, but don't forget your Little snacks!

Whether you're going to school, or staying at home, as you're doing your normal daily schedule I want you to take several breaks throughout the day to refuel with a glass of water and a small snack. These snacks should specifically remind you of Little Me. Some suggestions include: goldfish crackers, animal crackers, cheese cubes, lunchables, cheerios, etc.

Task #5: Stretch those muscles for 20 minutes of exercise!

This act of self-care will keep you feeling good and your body strong. Pick an activity that you already enjoy doing and exercise for 20 minutes.

Task #6: Evening D/s Movie

Every day for the next 25 days I want you to watch a movie that I've hand-picked that is designed to make you think about qualities that dominants should have. Characters in these movies all portray traits that most dom's exude. Think about the relationship dynamics and then follow up in Task #6 with your evening journal reflection letter.

Tonight's D/s Movie is: *The Edge of Seventeen (2016)*

Task #7: Evening Journal Reflection

Now that your day is starting to wind down and you have completed your first D/s movie, I want you to do an evening journal reflection. Instead of a typical diary entry, I want you to write a letter to your future dominant. You can begin by saying: Dear Future Dom... or Dear Dominant... or Dear Daddy/Mommy.... write what feels natural to you. Think about the qualities you want your dominant to have. Write about wishes you hope for, and dates you want to do with them. Write about the movie you watched tonight and things that are going on in your life. This journal will be a special gift to give your dom when you finally come together.

Task #8: Complete Your Night Time Routine
- Drink 1 glass of water

- Brush your teeth
- Turn off all social media and computers. Power down for the night.
- Pull on fresh pajamas
- If you have a picture book, (or checked one out from the library), lay down in bed and quietly read your book. If you don't have a picture book, listen to a read aloud picture book on YouTube. (There are bunches of videos!)
- Reduce your room lighting to a simple side lamp or fairy lights. Quiet the mind.
- Turn on soft lullaby music or classical music on YouTube
- As you begin to feel groggy, turn everything off, snuggle up to your plushie and drift off to sleep. (Make sure to get those 7-8 hours of rest in!).

Day 5: Finding Your Little Fashion Style

I have always been a plus size little, but that hasn't been easy to accept. When we Google "DDLG" or "Dd/l" and look at images we are often flooded by girls in cute outfits who happen to be very slender. Their long, lean legs are clad in thigh high stockings complete with a cat face around the knee. Perhaps, they are dressed in a onesie and their stomach is so flat you could eat off of it like a tray. It's easy to be jealous. It's more difficult to find your own path and style and see what works for you. Today this is our goal. Use DDLG/LB Youtubers as inspiration but think about what clothing type resonates with *your* personality! What do you want to wear in little space? Do you enjoy sundresses or pants? Do you want to wear a onesie or shorts and a t-shirt? No matter what body shape you have there are little clothing shops to accommodate your needs.

Amazon is an excellent place for all of your adult baby needs. However, if you are a Little or Middle you will need to venture out and seek other retailers. Etsy is another great site to browse. Search for DDLG clothing and you'll find dozens of private shops where members of the community can create custom clothing for you and all of your little space desires! Shopping should be fun. This is a time for you to reflect your outside with the way you feel on the inside.

While the bulk of DDLG/LB material and products available is geared towards little girls, I want to take a moment and focus on little boys. You are special and unique just as much as Little girls! As you continue your training like a good Little boy, I want you to think about what fashion style you see for yourself. Do you like graphic t-shirts with dinosaurs or Superman? (Target and Kohl's are excellent retailers to carry t-shirts of this kind). Would you like to wear denim overalls and a cute hat? Amazon carries denim overalls in your size that can easily make you feel like the good, Little boy that you are! Littleforbig also has an excellent selection of onesies that range from small up to 4XL and can accommodate any body type. Another idea is to search for light up sneakers for adults that you can wear that is discreetly Little, or you can invest in some adult AB diapers to wear under your normal street clothes that will make you feel Little without others seeing you in Little space. Get creative with your style and have fun with it!

After you've explored shopping and created your "wish list", turn your attention to your day 5 tasks.

Day 5 Tasks:

Task #1: Complete Your Morning Routine
- Drink 1 glass of water as soon as you wake up
- Wash your face
- Brush your teeth
- Throw your shower towel into the dryer (if available) and have it tumbling on low-medium heat while you hop into the shower.

- Shower up. While in the shower, think of a song you used to love as a child. Sing that song to yourself as you lather up. Then wrap yourself up in your warm towel afterward. Ahhh...
- Take time to pick out an outfit that is both comfortable, yet makes you feel pretty.
- Put on sunscreen and Chapstick
- Lotion your skin with baby lotion

Task #2: Meditate for 15 minutes

If you have a phone, I want you to download the FREE app. Headspace. It has guided meditation apps that are picked by the program based upon your current mood. If you do not have a phone, go onto YouTube and follow a 15-minute guided meditation video. Allow your breathing to calm and relax your body. Let go of your stresses and fears. Simply be. This daily practice is designed to train you to build up patience in sitting still as you will need to do for your dominant in the future.

Task #3: Browse DDLG/LB Fashion Online

Begin browsing fashion online to formulate your own unique little style! You can also see previous chapters (III., IV., and V. in this book for product and clothing suggestions). There is a style for everyone. Go and find yours!

Task #4: Time to start your normal day, but don't forget your Little snacks!

Whether you're going to school, or staying at home, as you're doing your normal daily schedule I want you to take several breaks throughout the day to refuel with a glass of water and a small snack. These snacks should specifically remind you of Little Me. Some suggestions include: goldfish crackers, animal crackers, cheese cubes, lunchables, cheerios, etc.

Task #5: Stretch those muscles for 20 minutes of exercise!

This act of self-care will keep you feeling good and your body strong. Pick an activity that you already enjoy doing and exercise for 20 minutes.

Task #6: Evening D/s Movie

Every day for the next 25 days I want you to watch a movie that I've hand-picked that is designed to make you think about qualities that dominants should have. Characters in these movies all portray traits that most dom's exude. Think about the relationship dynamics and then follow up in Task #6 with your evening journal reflection letter.

Tonight's D/s Movie is: *Noble, My Love (2015), a Korean TV series on Netflix with strong D/s themes.*

Task #7: Evening Journal Reflection

Now that your day is starting to wind down and you have completed your first D/s movie, I want you to do an evening journal reflection. Instead of a typical diary entry, I want you to write a letter to your future dominant. You can begin by saying: Dear Future Dom... or Dear Dominant... or Dear Daddy/Mommy.... write what feels natural to you. Think about the qualities you want your dominant to have. Write about wishes you hope for, and dates you want to do with them. Write about the movie you watched tonight and things that are going on in your life. This journal will be a special gift to give your dom when you finally come together.

Task #8: Complete Your Night Time Routine
- Drink 1 glass of water
- Brush your teeth
- Turn off all social media and computers. Power down for the night.
- Pull on fresh pajamas
- If you have a picture book, (or checked one out from the library), lay down in bed and quietly read your book. If you don't have a picture book, listen to a read aloud picture book on YouTube. (There are bunches of videos!)
- Reduce your room lighting to a simple side lamp or fairy lights. Quiet the mind.
- Turn on soft lullaby music or classical music on YouTube
- As you begin to feel groggy, turn everything off, snuggle up to your plushie and drift off to sleep. (Make sure to get those 7-8 hours of rest in!).

Day 6: Creating a Little Play Space

Welcome to Day 6 of your Little Training! Today we are going to get creative and dive into creating a physical play space for your living area. Some people are blessed with a spare bedroom to create an entire nursery. However, as someone who wasn't, I had to quickly learn how to make a Little space with a tiny amount of square feet. And now I'm going to show you how to do it too! Creating a Little space can seem overwhelming and intimidating especially if you are living at home with your parents, share a dorm or room with siblings, or you haven't quite decided if you *are* a Little. However, here are a few tips that you can do to minimize your stress while still creating a little play space to call your own:

- **Get an under the bed storage bin:** If you're sharing a bedroom or dorm space but still want to create a Little play space, try purchasing an under the bed storage bin. You can keep your toys and onesies in a discreet space to pull out whenever you are alone.
- **Remember less is more:** While you're creating your space, remember that it's not about the quantity of Little stuff you own, it's about purchasing items that move you into a little headspace. A simple plushie or watching free videos on YouTube of your favorite childhood shows can be all that it takes to make you slip into Little space.
- **Don't scar the vanilla peeps:** One rule that you'll often hear within the BDSM community is to never "scar" or show off your kink in front of a vanilla person. In other words, don't walk around in a onesie at the grocery store which forces non-DD/l people to see you in Little space. If you're living at home with family, "coming out" to them as a Little might be difficult and not something you're comfortable with. Wait until you are behind closed doors in the privacy of your own room to slip into Little space.
- **Go out and find Little friends:** If you don't have the ability to create a Little space within your home... go out and practice in a safe space outside of it! There are many DD/l conventions and meet up groups where you can make friends with other Littles (whether you have a daddy/mommy or not!). Some of the largest conventions and meet ups are as follows:
    1. CAPCon https://chicagoageplayers.com/
    2. Teddy Con http://www.teddycon.org/
    3. TOMKAT https://tomkatcamp.ca/
    4. West Coast Jungle Gym https://thewestcoastjunglegym.com/
    5. The Little Scouts http://www.thelittlescouts.com/

As well as online forums for you to chat and meet other Littles and dominants, including:
    1. DDLG Forum: https://www.ddlgforum.com/forum/4-little-space/
    2. ADISC.org The AB/ DL/ IC Support Community: https://www.adisc.org/forum/index.php

If you do have an extra bedroom or the privacy of your own room, then the world is your oyster in how you create your little space. You can hang a mobile over your bed or paint the walls in your favorite color. You can shop your local thrift stores and easily load up the space with fun toys and a play mat for all of your little space needs. Pinterest and Instagram are great places to view pictures of Little nurseries to give you inspiration for your own!

Now that you've got your creative juices flowing and have begun brainstorming how to design your own Little play space, let's turn our attention to your tasks for day 6.

Day 6 Tasks:

Task #1: Complete Your Morning Routine
- Drink 1 glass of water as soon as you wake up
- Wash your face
- Brush your teeth
- Throw your shower towel into the dryer (if available) and have it tumbling on low-medium heat while you hop into the shower.
- Shower up. While in the shower, think of a song you used to love as a child. Sing that song to yourself as you lather up. Then wrap yourself up in your warm towel afterward. Ahhh...
- Take time to pick out an outfit that is both comfortable, yet makes you feel pretty.
- Put on sunscreen and Chapstick
- Lotion your skin with baby lotion

Task #2: Meditate for 15 minutes
If you have a phone, I want you to download the FREE app. Headspace. It has guided meditation apps that are picked by the program based upon your current mood. If you do not have a phone, go onto YouTube and follow a 15-minute guided meditation video. Allow your breathing to calm and relax your body. Let go of your stresses and fears. Simply be. This daily practice is designed to train you to build up patience in sitting still as you will need to do for your dominant in the future.

Task #3: Browse DDLG/LB Fashion Online
Begin browsing fashion online to formulate your own unique little style! You can also see previous chapters (III., IV., and V. in this book for product and clothing suggestions). There is a style for everyone. Go and find yours!

Task #4: Time to start your normal day, but don't forget your Little snacks!
Whether you're going to school, or staying at home, as you're doing your normal daily schedule I want you to take several breaks throughout the day to refuel with a glass of water and a small snack. These snacks should specifically remind you of Little Me. Some suggestions include: goldfish crackers, animal crackers, cheese cubes, lunchables, cheerios, etc.

Task #5: Stretch those muscles for 20 minutes of exercise!
This act of self-care will keep you feeling good and your body strong. Pick an activity that you already enjoy doing and exercise for 20 minutes.

Task #6: Evening D/s Movie

Every day for the next 25 days I want you to watch a movie that I've hand-picked that is designed to make you think about qualities that dominants should have. Characters in these movies all portray traits that most dom's exude. Think about the relationship dynamics and then follow up in Task #6 with your evening journal reflection letter.

Tonight's D/s Movie is: *The Princess Diaries (2001)*

Task #7: Evening Journal Reflection

Now that your day is starting to wind down and you have completed your first D/s movie, I want you to do an evening journal reflection. Instead of a typical diary entry, I want you to write a letter to your future dominant. You can begin by saying: Dear Future Dom... or Dear Dominant... or Dear Daddy/Mommy.... write what feels natural to you. Think about the qualities you want your dominant to have. Write about wishes you hope for, and dates you want to do with them. Write about the movie you watched tonight and things that are going on in your life. This journal will be a special gift to give your dom when you finally come together.

Task #8: Complete Your Night Time Routine
- Drink 1 glass of water
- Brush your teeth
- Turn off all social media and computers. Power down for the night.
- Pull on fresh pajamas
- If you have a picture book, (or checked one out from the library), lay down in bed and quietly read your book. If you don't have a picture book, listen to a read aloud picture book on YouTube. (There are bunches of videos!)
- Reduce your room lighting to a simple side lamp or fairy lights. Quiet the mind.
- Turn on soft lullaby music or classical music on YouTube
- As you begin to feel groggy, turn everything off, snuggle up to your plushie and drift off to sleep. (Make sure to get those 7-8 hours of rest in!).

Day 7: Unearthing Your Childhood Passions

Welcome to Day 7 of your Little Training! Today we will focus on bringing to mind all of the favorite activities you used to love to do as a child. There is an old saying that what you wanted to be when you grew up when you were a child, is your true passion. If that's the case, then I need to get into the ice cream parlor business now. However, I do think there is truth to delving into your old childhood passions because it evokes a sense of serenity and calm within. Childhood passions are often activities that make you feel good, involve movement, and leave you without a care in the world. What were your favorite things to do as a child?

For this exercise, begin by taking out a blank sheet of paper and a pen. Without much thought, start writing down as many childhood activities that you used to love to do in a list on the page. Don't think too much, just write what comes to mind first. This is your brain's way of unearthing your true passions, the things that made you genuinely happy at that point in time. Smile. Bask in the memories of your youth. When you've completed your list, go back over and look at everything you've written. Cross out any activities that you know instantly that you would never want to do again. Then reevaluate your list. Circle any items that are things you wish to do again. Take all of the circles and turn them into a separate list. Now you have a list of little activities to pursue!

Reflect on how these little activities make you feel. Are you excited to try them again? Are you nervous? Be sure to journal your feelings down in your evening journal reflection letter. For now, let's look at your day 7 tasks.

Day 7 Tasks:

Task #1: Complete Your Morning Routine
- Drink 1 glass of water as soon as you wake up
- Wash your face
- Brush your teeth
- Throw your shower towel into the dryer (if available) and have it tumbling on low-medium heat while you hop into the shower.
- Shower up. While in the shower, think of a song you used to love as a child. Sing that song to yourself as you lather up. Then wrap yourself up in your warm towel afterward. Ahhh...
- Take time to pick out an outfit that is both comfortable, yet makes you feel pretty.
- Put on sunscreen and Chapstick
- Lotion your skin with baby lotion

Task #2: Meditate for 15 minutes
If you have a phone, I want you to download the FREE app. Headspace. It has guided meditation apps that are picked by the program based upon your current mood. If you do not have a phone, go onto YouTube and follow a 15-minute guided meditation video. Allow your breathing to calm and relax your

body. Let go of your stresses and fears. Simply be. This daily practice is designed to train you to build up patience in sitting still as you will need to do for your dominant in the future.

Task #3: Browse DDLG/LB Fashion Online

Begin browsing fashion online to formulate your own unique little style! You can also see previous chapters (III., IV., and V. in this book for product and clothing suggestions). There is a style for everyone. Go and find yours!

Task #4: Time to start your normal day, but don't forget your Little snacks!

Whether you're going to school, or staying at home, as you're doing your normal daily schedule I want you to take several breaks throughout the day to refuel with a glass of water and a small snack. These snacks should specifically remind you of Little Me. Some suggestions include: goldfish crackers, animal crackers, cheese cubes, lunchables, cheerios, etc.

Task #5: Stretch those muscles for 20 minutes of exercise!

This act of self-care will keep you feeling good and your body strong. Pick an activity that you already enjoy doing and exercise for 20 minutes.

Task #6: Evening D/s Movie

Every day for the next 25 days I want you to watch a movie that I've hand-picked that is designed to make you think about qualities that dominants should have. Characters in these movies all portray traits that most dom's exude. Think about the relationship dynamics and then follow up in Task #6 with your evening journal reflection letter.

Tonight's D/s Movie is: *She's The Man (2006)*

Task #7: Evening Journal Reflection

Now that your day is starting to wind down and you have completed your first D/s movie, I want you to do an evening journal reflection. Instead of a typical diary entry, I want you to write a letter to your future dominant. You can begin by saying: Dear Future Dom... or Dear Dominant... or Dear Daddy/Mommy.... write what feels natural to you. Think about the qualities you want your dominant to have. Write about wishes you hope for, and dates you want to do with them. Write about the movie you watched tonight and things that are going on in your life. This journal will be a special gift to give your dom when you finally come together.

Task #8: Complete Your Night Time Routine
- Drink 1 glass of water
- Brush your teeth
- Turn off all social media and computers. Power down for the night.
- Pull on fresh pajamas

- If you have a picture book, (or checked one out from the library), lay down in bed and quietly read your book. If you don't have a picture book, listen to a read aloud picture book on YouTube. (There are bunches of videos!)
- Reduce your room lighting to a simple side lamp or fairy lights. Quiet the mind.
- Turn on soft lullaby music or classical music on YouTube
- As you begin to feel groggy, turn everything off, snuggle up to your plushie and drift off to sleep. (Make sure to get those 7–8 hours of rest in!).

Day 8: Get Outside! Being a Little in Public

It can be a scary thing navigating the world as a Little. There are times when something will trigger you into little space while you're out in public. This is completely normal, but knowing how to handle yourself is key. As you grow comfortable in little space you might develop a separate tone or pattern of speech that you use only while being little. You might also take on other behaviors while in Little space such as: playing on the floor, getting more excited and energetic, or becoming non-verbal and only conveying your needs with behavior and emotions (as in regressing to infancy). Here are a few tips to remember while being little in public:

- **Keep the noise down:** It's fine to be Little in public and you can do so discreetly as long as you aren't too loud. Don't draw attention to yourself if you don't need to.
- **Change Your Pet Names:** If you are hanging out with other Littles, you might want to use your "adult" name versus your pet/little name to keep things more discreet.
- **Opt for childlike street wear:** There are many clothing items that can make you feel little without being overtly DDLG/LB. (Think overalls).

Your Challenge For Today: Choose an outfit that makes you feel Little and happy. Wear something comfortable and then take a walk. If you have a nearby park or playground, play on the playground for a few minutes. If not, take a walk and simply enjoy nature. Allow your mind to regress into little space as you take in the world around you. Enjoy being Little in public, while still keeping your privacy!

And now let's take a look at your day 8 tasks:

Day 8 Tasks:

Task #1: Complete Your Morning Routine
- Drink 1 glass of water as soon as you wake up
- Wash your face
- Brush your teeth
- Throw your shower towel into the dryer (if available) and have it tumbling on low-medium heat while you hop into the shower.
- Shower up. While in the shower, think of a song you used to love as a child. Sing that song to yourself as you lather up. Then wrap yourself up in your warm towel afterward. Ahhh...
- Take time to pick out an outfit that is both comfortable, yet makes you feel pretty.
- Put on sunscreen and Chapstick
- Lotion your skin with baby lotion

Task #2: Meditate for 15 minutes
If you have a phone, I want you to download the FREE app. Headspace. It has guided meditation apps that are picked by the program based upon your current mood. If you do not have a phone, go onto YouTube and follow a 15-minute guided meditation video. Allow your breathing to calm and relax your

body. Let go of your stresses and fears. Simply be. This daily practice is designed to train you to build up patience in sitting still as you will need to do for your dominant in the future.

Task #3: Browse DDLG/LB Fashion Online

Begin browsing fashion online to formulate your own unique little style! You can also see previous chapters (III., IV., and V. in this book for product and clothing suggestions). There is a style for everyone. Go and find yours!

Task #4: Time to start your normal day, but don't forget your Little snacks!

Whether you're going to school, or staying at home, as you're doing your normal daily schedule I want you to take several breaks throughout the day to refuel with a glass of water and a small snack. These snacks should specifically remind you of Little Me. Some suggestions include: goldfish crackers, animal crackers, cheese cubes, lunchables, cheerios, etc.

Task #5: Stretch those muscles for 20 minutes of exercise!

This act of self-care will keep you feeling good and your body strong. Pick an activity that you already enjoy doing and exercise for 20 minutes.

Task #6: Evening D/s Movie

Every day for the next 25 days I want you to watch a movie that I've hand-picked that is designed to make you think about qualities that dominants should have. Characters in these movies all portray traits that most dom's exude. Think about the relationship dynamics and then follow up in Task #6 with your evening journal reflection letter.

Tonight's D/s Movie is: *13 Going On 30 (2004)*

Task #7: Evening Journal Reflection

Now that your day is starting to wind down and you have completed your first D/s movie, I want you to do an evening journal reflection. Instead of a typical diary entry, I want you to write a letter to your future dominant. You can begin by saying: Dear Future Dom... or Dear Dominant... or Dear Daddy/Mommy.... write what feels natural to you. Think about the qualities you want your dominant to have. Write about wishes you hope for, and dates you want to do with them. Write about the movie you watched tonight and things that are going on in your life. This journal will be a special gift to give your dom when you finally come together.

Task #8: Complete Your Night Time Routine
- Drink 1 glass of water
- Brush your teeth
- Turn off all social media and computers. Power down for the night.
- Pull on fresh pajamas

- If you have a picture book, (or checked one out from the library), lay down in bed and quietly read your book. If you don't have a picture book, listen to a read aloud picture book on YouTube. (There are bunches of videos!)
- Reduce your room lighting to a simple side lamp or fairy lights. Quiet the mind.
- Turn on soft lullaby music or classical music on YouTube
- As you begin to feel groggy, turn everything off, snuggle up to your plushie and drift off to sleep. (Make sure to get those 7-8 hours of rest in!).

Day 9: Nurturing Within: Seeing Your True Beauty

I would be remiss if I said that there wasn't some visual aspect to being a little. A dominant relies on their Little dressing like a Little, acting like a Little, and really getting into Little space full on. It is a suspension of the mind on both parties. However, that said, a dominant should never, ever judge you based upon your appearance. You are beautiful! Today is going to focus on how you see yourself versus how the world sees you. Often times we are the most critical person of ourselves. We judge ourselves harshly because we feel like the world is doing so, but that isn't necessarily the case. In fact, many times people will find you pretty and attractive. Having a low self-esteem not only impairs your mental health, but it can deter a dominant from bonding with you. Take heart, my fellow Little-friend! There is a dominant out there for you. You just have to believe in yourself!

Today's Challenge: Gather a cell phone or camera and take a picture of yourself. No, I'm not asking for you to pose for the perfect selfie. You don't need to do that silly, downward angle-thing in which it supposedly makes you look slimmer, when in reality everyone knows that you're trying to get that exact angle. No. I want you to snap a picture as you are. Hold up the camera and just click. Then, before you look at the picture, gather a piece of paper and some crayons, markers, etc. and draw a picture of yourself **as you see yourself.** When you've finished, compare your drawing with the picture you took with your camera. What qualities were different? What were the same? Did you accentuate features of yours and were they represented accurately or not?

Reflect on how you feel. The next time you think of yourself, remember this exercise. You are *far* more beautiful than you think you are! Love yourself, because you're worth it my friend. And now let's turn our attention to your day 9 tasks.

Day 9 Tasks:

Task #1: Complete Your Morning Routine
- Drink 1 glass of water as soon as you wake up
- Wash your face
- Brush your teeth
- Throw your shower towel into the dryer (if available) and have it tumbling on low-medium heat while you hop into the shower.
- Shower up. While in the shower, think of a song you used to love as a child. Sing that song to yourself as you lather up. Then wrap yourself up in your warm towel afterward. Ahhh...
- Take time to pick out an outfit that is both comfortable, yet makes you feel pretty.
- Put on sunscreen and Chapstick
- Lotion your skin with baby lotion

Task #2: Meditate for 15 minutes

If you have a phone, I want you to download the FREE app. Headspace. It has guided meditation apps that are picked by the program based upon your current mood. If you do not have a phone, go onto YouTube and follow a 15-minute guided meditation video. Allow your breathing to calm and relax your body. Let go of your stresses and fears. Simply be. This daily practice is designed to train you to build up patience in sitting still as you will need to do for your dominant in the future.

Task #3: Browse DDLG/LB Fashion Online

Begin browsing fashion online to formulate your own unique little style! You can also see previous chapters (III., IV., and V. in this book for product and clothing suggestions). There is a style for everyone. Go and find yours!

Task #4: Time to start your normal day, but don't forget your Little snacks!

Whether you're going to school, or staying at home, as you're doing your normal daily schedule I want you to take several breaks throughout the day to refuel with a glass of water and a small snack. These snacks should specifically remind you of Little Me. Some suggestions include: goldfish crackers, animal crackers, cheese cubes, lunchables, cheerios, etc.

Task #5: Stretch those muscles for 20 minutes of exercise!

This act of self-care will keep you feeling good and your body strong. Pick an activity that you already enjoy doing and exercise for 20 minutes.

Task #6: Evening D/s Movie

Every day for the next 25 days I want you to watch a movie that I've hand-picked that is designed to make you think about qualities that dominants should have. Characters in these movies all portray traits that most dom's exude. Think about the relationship dynamics and then follow up in Task #6 with your evening journal reflection letter.

Tonight's D/s Movie is: *Penelope (2007)*

Task #7: Evening Journal Reflection

Now that your day is starting to wind down and you have completed your first D/s movie, I want you to do an evening journal reflection. Instead of a typical diary entry, I want you to write a letter to your future dominant. You can begin by saying: Dear Future Dom... or Dear Dominant... or Dear Daddy/Mommy.... write what feels natural to you. Think about the qualities you want your dominant to have. Write about wishes you hope for, and dates you want to do with them. Write about the movie you watched tonight and things that are going on in your life. This journal will be a special gift to give your dom when you finally come together.

Task #8: Complete Your Night Time Routine

- Drink 1 glass of water
- Brush your teeth

- Turn off all social media and computers. Power down for the night.
- Pull on fresh pajamas
- If you have a picture book, (or checked one out from the library), lay down in bed and quietly read your book. If you don't have a picture book, listen to a read aloud picture book on YouTube. (There are bunches of videos!)
- Reduce your room lighting to a simple side lamp or fairy lights. Quiet the mind.
- Turn on soft lullaby music or classical music on YouTube
- As you begin to feel groggy, turn everything off, snuggle up to your plushie and drift off to sleep. (Make sure to get those 7-8 hours of rest in!).

Day 10: Self-Care: An at Home Spa-- Little Style!

Welcome to Day 10 of your Little Training! Today I want to talk about self-care and ways in which you can turn a normal day into a Little retreat by pampering yourself. If you've never been to a spa, you have to go once. Just once is enough, because (and I'm keeping it real here!) a spa can be a pricey trip. Since I haven't figured out how to grow a money tree (when I do, I'll tell you), we must bring the spa home to pamper ourselves! There are many DIY spa recipes online for you to explore, but for today we will focus on your face. Why? Because the face is the very first thing that most people notice.

You don't need to go investing in a ton of masks, creams, serums, and whatever else is out there on the market, to get a flawless face. Instead, walk into the kitchen and grab two ingredients: oatmeal and honey. Preferably you want to use cheap, quick oats but old-fashioned works fine too. Mix 1 cup of oatmeal with 1 tablespoon of honey together. Add a bit of hot water into the bowl until it makes a paste and you're ready to go! Honey and oatmeal both have properties to cleanse and exfoliate your face while leaving it rejuvenated and it doesn't strip away vital hydration for your skin.

Here are some other ways to create an at-home spa:

- Give yourself a bubble bath
- Paint your nails (and toenails too!)
- Rub baby lotion on your skin or put baby powder on your body after your bath
- Play around with makeup
- Put on body glitter and make yourself sparkle!
- Purchase some facial rose water spray on Amazon ($7 USD) and give your face a spritz to rejuvenate your senses

Your Challenge For Today: Create a facial scrub with the above recipe and use some of the tips listed to give yourself an at home spa day. Relax your body and your mind as you let go.

After you've completed your challenge, move on to your day 10 tasks.

Day 10 Tasks:

Task #1: Complete Your Morning Routine
- Drink 1 glass of water as soon as you wake up
- Wash your face
- Brush your teeth
- Throw your shower towel into the dryer (if available) and have it tumbling on low-medium heat while you hop into the shower.
- Shower up. While in the shower, think of a song you used to love as a child. Sing that song to yourself as you lather up. Then wrap yourself up in your warm towel afterward. Ahhh...
- Take time to pick out an outfit that is both comfortable, yet makes you feel pretty.
- Put on sunscreen and Chapstick

- Lotion your skin with baby lotion

Task #2: Meditate for 15 minutes

If you have a phone, I want you to download the FREE app. Headspace. It has guided meditation apps that are picked by the program based upon your current mood. If you do not have a phone, go onto YouTube and follow a 15-minute guided meditation video. Allow your breathing to calm and relax your body. Let go of your stresses and fears. Simply be. This daily practice is designed to train you to build up patience in sitting still as you will need to do for your dominant in the future.

Task #3: Browse DDLG/LB Fashion Online

Begin browsing fashion online to formulate your own unique little style! You can also see previous chapters (III., IV., and V. in this book for product and clothing suggestions). There is a style for everyone. Go and find yours!

Task #4: Time to start your normal day, but don't forget your Little snacks!

Whether you're going to school, or staying at home, as you're doing your normal daily schedule I want you to take several breaks throughout the day to refuel with a glass of water and a small snack. These snacks should specifically remind you of Little Me. Some suggestions include: goldfish crackers, animal crackers, cheese cubes, lunchables, cheerios, etc.

Task #5: Stretch those muscles for 20 minutes of exercise!

This act of self-care will keep you feeling good and your body strong. Pick an activity that you already enjoy doing and exercise for 20 minutes.

Task #6: Evening D/s Movie

Every day for the next 25 days I want you to watch a movie that I've hand-picked that is designed to make you think about qualities that dominants should have. Characters in these movies all portray traits that most dom's exude. Think about the relationship dynamics and then follow up in Task #6 with your evening journal reflection letter.

Tonight's D/s Movie is: *Mulan (1998)*

Task #7: Evening Journal Reflection

Now that your day is starting to wind down and you have completed your first D/s movie, I want you to do an evening journal reflection. Instead of a typical diary entry, I want you to write a letter to your future dominant. You can begin by saying: Dear Future Dom... or Dear Dominant... or Dear Daddy/Mommy.... write what feels natural to you. Think about the qualities you want your dominant to have. Write about wishes you hope for, and dates you want to do with them. Write about the movie you watched tonight and things that are going on in your life. This journal will be a special gift to give your dom when you finally come together.

Task #8: Complete Your Night Time Routine
- Drink 1 glass of water
- Brush your teeth
- Turn off all social media and computers. Power down for the night.
- Pull on fresh pajamas
- If you have a picture book, (or checked one out from the library), lay down in bed and quietly read your book. If you don't have a picture book, listen to a read aloud picture book on YouTube. (There are bunches of videos!)
- Reduce your room lighting to a simple side lamp or fairy lights. Quiet the mind.
- Turn on soft lullaby music or classical music on YouTube
- As you begin to feel groggy, turn everything off, snuggle up to your plushie and drift off to sleep. (Make sure to get those 7-8 hours of rest in!).

Day 11: Little Nibbles: Testing Out Fun, Little Foods

Part of becoming a Little is experiencing Little space no matter what you're doing. Eating or having a snack is no exception. I included having a Little snack in your daily tasks to help you feel Little while you're out in your normal, everyday schedule. Today we will focus on foods that you can purchase in the grocery store to make you feel more Little while eating at home. Little foods are all about portion sizes. Nothing screams Little food more than tiny bites or adorable colors. There are plenty of "child-themed" foods available for purchase. Your challenge today is simple: pick and choose as many Little foods as possible from the grocery store and taste test which ones you enjoy. Keep a list somewhere (or paper or in your phone) of which ones you enjoy. Then refer back to that list on your weekly grocery trip so you always have Little foods on hand to use in Little space. Here are some suggestions to get you thinking:

- Goldfish (rainbow or baby ones!)
- Animal crackers
- Mickey Mouse frozen Toaster Waffles
- Hot Pockets
- Lunchables
- Snack Pack Pudding Cups
- Gummi packs
- Kid-cuisine frozen entree meals
- Bagel bites
- Cheerios
- Funfetti cake box mix and Funfetti icing
- Bento box recipes
- Chicken nuggets (or dino nuggets)
- Waffle fries
- Individual ice cream cups
- Go-gurt, squeezable yogurt tubes
- Squeezable/suck-able applesauce packets
- Apple slice packs
- Boxed macaroni and cheese with special noodle shapes
- Berry and cream cups (check your local produce section)
- Keebler Elf Cookies
- Smuckers or Tropical Peanut Butter & Jelly Twist Jar

When you have completed your challenge, please move on to your day 11 tasks.

Day 11 Tasks:

Task #1: Complete Your Morning Routine

- Drink 1 glass of water as soon as you wake up
- Wash your face
- Brush your teeth
- Throw your shower towel into the dryer (if available) and have it tumbling on low-medium heat while you hop into the shower.
- Shower up. While in the shower, think of a song you used to love as a child. Sing that song to yourself as you lather up. Then wrap yourself up in your warm towel afterward. Ahhh...
- Take time to pick out an outfit that is both comfortable, yet makes you feel pretty.
- Put on sunscreen and Chapstick
- Lotion your skin with baby lotion

Task #2: Meditate for 15 minutes

If you have a phone, I want you to download the FREE app. Headspace. It has guided meditation apps that are picked by the program based upon your current mood. If you do not have a phone, go onto YouTube and follow a 15-minute guided meditation video. Allow your breathing to calm and relax your body. Let go of your stresses and fears. Simply be. This daily practice is designed to train you to build up patience in sitting still as you will need to do for your dominant in the future.

Task #3: Browse DDLG/LB Fashion Online

Begin browsing fashion online to formulate your own unique little style! You can also see previous chapters (III., IV., and V. in this book for product and clothing suggestions). There is a style for everyone. Go and find yours!

Task #4: Time to start your normal day, but don't forget your Little snacks!

Whether you're going to school, or staying at home, as you're doing your normal daily schedule I want you to take several breaks throughout the day to refuel with a glass of water and a small snack. These snacks should specifically remind you of Little Me. Some suggestions include: goldfish crackers, animal crackers, cheese cubes, lunchables, cheerios, etc.

Task #5: Stretch those muscles for 20 minutes of exercise!

This act of self-care will keep you feeling good and your body strong. Pick an activity that you already enjoy doing and exercise for 20 minutes.

Task #6: Evening D/s Movie

Every day for the next 25 days I want you to watch a movie that I've hand-picked that is designed to make you think about qualities that dominants should have. Characters in these movies all portray traits that most dom's exude. Think about the relationship dynamics and then follow up in Task #6 with your evening journal reflection letter.

Tonight's D/s Movie is: *Beauty and the Beast (2017)*

Task #7: Evening Journal Reflection

Now that your day is starting to wind down and you have completed your first D/s movie, I want you to do an evening journal reflection. Instead of a typical diary entry, I want you to write a letter to your future dominant. You can begin by saying: Dear Future Dom... or Dear Dominant... or Dear Daddy/Mommy.... write what feels natural to you. Think about the qualities you want your dominant to have. Write about wishes you hope for, and dates you want to do with them. Write about the movie you watched tonight and things that are going on in your life. This journal will be a special gift to give your dom when you finally come together.

Task #8: Complete Your Night Time Routine
- Drink 1 glass of water
- Brush your teeth
- Turn off all social media and computers. Power down for the night.
- Pull on fresh pajamas
- If you have a picture book, (or checked one out from the library), lay down in bed and quietly read your book. If you don't have a picture book, listen to a read aloud picture book on YouTube. (There are bunches of videos!)
- Reduce your room lighting to a simple side lamp or fairy lights. Quiet the mind.
- Turn on soft lullaby music or classical music on YouTube
- As you begin to feel groggy, turn everything off, snuggle up to your plushie and drift off to sleep. (Make sure to get those 7-8 hours of rest in!).

Day 12: Silence is Golden & The Art of Meditation

If there is one thing that Littles struggle with, it's patience! Generally speaking, when a Little is in Little space, they don't have very much patience at all. Although it should be noted that having a lack of patience and a lack of respect are two entirely different things. It's one thing to get impatient while waiting your turn for a toy at a convention. It's another to whine or throw a tantrum at another Little while waiting to use said toy.

By now you've been meditating for 15 minutes per day, so you're probably a pro at this! Sitting still is an important task because your future dominant will want to snuggle with you, or have you sit next to them quietly as they do their own work. Having the ability to sit still is an important lesson to learn, so today your task is to meditate in silence without the use of a guided meditation video. If you have to have one playing, then of course that's fine. But if possible, try sitting in absolute silence for 15 minutes and just be. If your mind wanders, gently bring it back to present. Be still within yourself as you slowly train your body to be present where you are. You're doing so well! When your 15-minute meditation has been completed, please move onto your day 12 tasks.

Day 12 Tasks:

Task #1: Complete Your Morning Routine
- Drink 1 glass of water as soon as you wake up
- Wash your face
- Brush your teeth
- Throw your shower towel into the dryer (if available) and have it tumbling on low-medium heat while you hop into the shower.
- Shower up. While in the shower, think of a song you used to love as a child. Sing that song to yourself as you lather up. Then wrap yourself up in your warm towel afterward. Ahhh...
- Take time to pick out an outfit that is both comfortable, yet makes you feel pretty.
- Put on sunscreen and Chapstick
- Lotion your skin with baby lotion

Task #2: Meditate for 15 minutes
If you have a phone, I want you to download the FREE app. Headspace. It has guided meditation apps that are picked by the program based upon your current mood. If you do not have a phone, go onto YouTube and follow a 15-minute guided meditation video. Allow your breathing to calm and relax your body. Let go of your stresses and fears. Simply be. This daily practice is designed to train you to build up patience in sitting still as you will need to do for your dominant in the future.

Task #3: Browse DDLG/LB Fashion Online

Begin browsing fashion online to formulate your own unique little style! You can also see previous chapters (III., IV., and V. in this book for product and clothing suggestions). There is a style for everyone. Go and find yours!

Task #4: Time to start your normal day, but don't forget your Little snacks!

Whether you're going to school, or staying at home, as you're doing your normal daily schedule I want you to take several breaks throughout the day to refuel with a glass of water and a small snack. These snacks should specifically remind you of Little Me. Some suggestions include: goldfish crackers, animal crackers, cheese cubes, lunchables, cheerios, etc.

Task #5: Stretch those muscles for 20 minutes of exercise!

This act of self-care will keep you feeling good and your body strong. Pick an activity that you already enjoy doing and exercise for 20 minutes.

Task #6: Evening D/s Movie

Every day for the next 25 days I want you to watch a movie that I've hand-picked that is designed to make you think about qualities that dominants should have. Characters in these movies all portray traits that most dom's exude. Think about the relationship dynamics and then follow up in Task #6 with your evening journal reflection letter.

Tonight's D/s Movie is: *Pocahontas (1995)*

Task #7: Evening Journal Reflection

Now that your day is starting to wind down and you have completed your first D/s movie, I want you to do an evening journal reflection. Instead of a typical diary entry, I want you to write a letter to your future dominant. You can begin by saying: Dear Future Dom... or Dear Dominant... or Dear Daddy/Mommy.... write what feels natural to you. Think about the qualities you want your dominant to have. Write about wishes you hope for, and dates you want to do with them. Write about the movie you watched tonight and things that are going on in your life. This journal will be a special gift to give your dom when you finally come together.

Task #8: Complete Your Night Time Routine

- Drink 1 glass of water
- Brush your teeth
- Turn off all social media and computers. Power down for the night.
- Pull on fresh pajamas
- If you have a picture book, (or checked one out from the library), lay down in bed and quietly read your book. If you don't have a picture book, listen to a read aloud picture book on YouTube. (There are bunches of videos!)
- Reduce your room lighting to a simple side lamp or fairy lights. Quiet the mind.
- Turn on soft lullaby music or classical music on YouTube

- As you begin to feel groggy, turn everything off, snuggle up to your plushie and drift off to sleep. (Make sure to get those 7-8 hours of rest in!).

Day 13: Rediscovering Pretend Play

Welcome to Day 13 of Little Training! Today's focus will be opening up your mind to rediscovering pretend play. Using your imagination requires an open mind. You can't expect to transform an ordinary stick into a magical wand without suspending your mind and really believing that the stick *is* a wand. Turning the world around you into a magical paradise takes faith, trust, (and a little bit of pixie dust!) and your imagination. An ordinary rock can be painted with a face to become a troll-friend. A walk in the park suddenly turns into an adventure into an elven woodland. A swim at the pool opens your mind to becoming a mermaid! You get the idea. You needn't feel silly or shy at using your imagination to bring a bit of magic into your life. All over the world people are starting to use their imagination to do all kinds of wonderful things.

- You can purchase mermaid tails to use as you swim in the pool.
- You can connect with a local LARPing (Live Action Role Playing) chapter and actually become a character. Participants dress up as their characters and go camping for the weekend to fight monsters with foam weapons and bean bags. (Visit: https://larping.org/)
- You can connect with the Society of Creative Anachronism, Inc. to get involved with a chapter that hosts Renaissance events. (Visit: http://www.sca.org/)
- You can even dress up as a pirate! (Visit: http://www.gentlemenoffortune.com/)
- Bedtime stories can be turned into a shadow puppet theater with nothing more than a flashlight and your hands
- You can have a tea party with your plushies with a stack of paper cups, some water or juice, and a snack.

There are numerous ways to make your world a bit more magical and play around with different personas. Yes, you are a little, but you may also want to be a wizard and attend Hogwarts. You may want to be an animal and dress up with ears and a tail. Let your mind wander and roam as you explore how to make your everyday life a bit more fun.

Your Challenge: Close your eyes and envision a scene that is magical and otherworldly. Maybe it's a scene from a movie you've watched, or perhaps it's something you've read in a book. Then open your eyes and see how you can bring that place to life with your imagination. Use every day props to transform into magical tools and spend at least 15 minutes in pretend play.

After you've completed your challenge, please move on to your day 13 tasks.

Day 13 Tasks:

Task #1: Complete Your Morning Routine
- Drink 1 glass of water as soon as you wake up
- Wash your face

- Brush your teeth
- Throw your shower towel into the dryer (if available) and have it tumbling on low-medium heat while you hop into the shower.
- Shower up. While in the shower, think of a song you used to love as a child. Sing that song to yourself as you lather up. Then wrap yourself up in your warm towel afterward. Ahhh...
- Take time to pick out an outfit that is both comfortable, yet makes you feel pretty.
- Put on sunscreen and Chapstick
- Lotion your skin with baby lotion

Task #2: Meditate for 15 minutes

If you have a phone, I want you to download the FREE app. Headspace. It has guided meditation apps that are picked by the program based upon your current mood. If you do not have a phone, go onto YouTube and follow a 15-minute guided meditation video. Allow your breathing to calm and relax your body. Let go of your stresses and fears. Simply be. This daily practice is designed to train you to build up patience in sitting still as you will need to do for your dominant in the future.

Task #3: Browse DDLG/LB Fashion Online

Begin browsing fashion online to formulate your own unique little style! You can also see previous chapters (III., IV., and V. in this book for product and clothing suggestions). There is a style for everyone. Go and find yours!

Task #4: Time to start your normal day, but don't forget your Little snacks!

Whether you're going to school, or staying at home, as you're doing your normal daily schedule I want you to take several breaks throughout the day to refuel with a glass of water and a small snack. These snacks should specifically remind you of Little Me. Some suggestions include: goldfish crackers, animal crackers, cheese cubes, lunchables, cheerios, etc.

Task #5: Stretch those muscles for 20 minutes of exercise!

This act of self-care will keep you feeling good and your body strong. Pick an activity that you already enjoy doing and exercise for 20 minutes.

Task #6: Evening D/s Movie

Every day for the next 25 days I want you to watch a movie that I've hand-picked that is designed to make you think about qualities that dominants should have. Characters in these movies all portray traits that most dom's exude. Think about the relationship dynamics and then follow up in Task #6 with your evening journal reflection letter.

Tonight's D/s Movie is: *A Christmas Prince (2017)*

Task #7: Evening Journal Reflection

Now that your day is starting to wind down and you have completed your first D/s movie, I want you to do an evening journal reflection. Instead of a typical diary entry, I want you to write a letter to your future dominant. You can begin by saying: Dear Future Dom... or Dear Dominant... or Dear Daddy/Mommy.... write what feels natural to you. Think about the qualities you want your dominant to have. Write about wishes you hope for, and dates you want to do with them. Write about the movie you watched tonight and things that are going on in your life. This journal will be a special gift to give your dom when you finally come together.

Task #8: Complete Your Night Time Routine
- Drink 1 glass of water
- Brush your teeth
- Turn off all social media and computers. Power down for the night.
- Pull on fresh pajamas
- If you have a picture book, (or checked one out from the library), lay down in bed and quietly read your book. If you don't have a picture book, listen to a read aloud picture book on YouTube. (There are bunches of videos!)
- Reduce your room lighting to a simple side lamp or fairy lights. Quiet the mind.
- Turn on soft lullaby music or classical music on YouTube
- As you begin to feel groggy, turn everything off, snuggle up to your plushie and drift off to sleep. (Make sure to get those 7-8 hours of rest in!).

Day 14: Getting Artsy in Little Space

Welcome to Day 14 of your Little Training! Today is all about getting messy and creating something beautiful as you spend time in Little space. If you've been chatting online and making some new little friends, this is the perfect time to show off your artwork by taking a picture and posting it on the online forum you like. One of the easiest, and best ways to slip into Little space is through arts and crafts. Below are some ideas for you to create something to enhance your Little play space while staying on a budget and having fun. Your challenge for today is to pick one craft off of the list below and complete it! Then enjoy the fruits of your labor the next time you slip into Little space! Now have fun and get crafting, my friend!

Your Challenge: Pick one arts and crafts task below and complete it to create a new item for your play space.

- Order an adult pacifier from Amazon ($7 USD) but make sure it is a blank one! When it arrives in the mail, decorate it with stickers or gems, however you'd like!
- Purchase a cheap mason jar from the store and paint the outside with your favorite colors. Use this (along with a mason jar nipple) the next time you want to bottle feed with a drink!
- Go to the craft store and pick up a blank, white t-shirt and craft markers or puffy paint. Create a new Little-inspired t-shirt to wear in little space.
- Go to a discount shoe store and pick out blank white slip on (or lace up shoes). Then get permanent colorful markers and have a blast drawing all over them with your favorite happy images.
- Go to your local craft store and pick up a bag of wooden peg dolls (blank). Next, grab some paints, markers, or whatever else you have on hand and create a set of dolls to play with that fit in the palm of your hand!
- Go to the craft store and pick up a bucket of colorful beads (some with letters and some not) and some lanyard. Make a bracelet to wear. (Maybe you want to use your little name on the bracelet?).
- Get a pack of washable finger paints and some art paper and let your little me shine as you get messy and make a pretty picture!

When you've completed your art project, please move on to your day 14 tasks.

Day 14 Tasks:

Task #1: Complete Your Morning Routine

- Drink 1 glass of water as soon as you wake up
- Wash your face
- Brush your teeth
- Throw your shower towel into the dryer (if available) and have it tumbling on low-medium heat while you hop into the shower.
- Shower up. While in the shower, think of a song you used to love as a child. Sing that song to yourself as you lather up. Then wrap yourself up in your warm towel afterward. Ahhh...
- Take time to pick out an outfit that is both comfortable, yet makes you feel pretty.
- Put on sunscreen and Chapstick
- Lotion your skin with baby lotion

Task #2: Meditate for 15 minutes

If you have a phone, I want you to download the FREE app. Headspace. It has guided meditation apps that are picked by the program based upon your current mood. If you do not have a phone, go onto YouTube and follow a 15-minute guided meditation video. Allow your breathing to calm and relax your body. Let go of your stresses and fears. Simply be. This daily practice is designed to train you to build up patience in sitting still as you will need to do for your dominant in the future.

Task #3: Browse DDLG/LB Fashion Online

Begin browsing fashion online to formulate your own unique little style! You can also see previous chapters (III., IV., and V. in this book for product and clothing suggestions). There is a style for everyone. Go and find yours!

Task #4: Time to start your normal day, but don't forget your Little snacks!

Whether you're going to school, or staying at home, as you're doing your normal daily schedule I want you to take several breaks throughout the day to refuel with a glass of water and a small snack. These snacks should specifically remind you of Little Me. Some suggestions include: goldfish crackers, animal crackers, cheese cubes, lunchables, cheerios, etc.

Task #5: Stretch those muscles for 20 minutes of exercise!

This act of self-care will keep you feeling good and your body strong. Pick an activity that you already enjoy doing and exercise for 20 minutes.

Task #6: Evening D/s Movie

Every day for the next 25 days I want you to watch a movie that I've hand-picked that is designed to make you think about qualities that dominants should have. Characters in these movies all portray traits that most dom's exude. Think about the relationship dynamics and then follow up in Task #6 with your evening journal reflection letter.

Tonight's D/s Movie is: *Spanglish (2004)*

Task #7: Evening Journal Reflection

Now that your day is starting to wind down and you have completed your first D/s movie, I want you to do an evening journal reflection. Instead of a typical diary entry, I want you to write a letter to your future dominant. You can begin by saying: Dear Future Dom... or Dear Dominant... or Dear Daddy/Mommy.... write what feels natural to you. Think about the qualities you want your dominant to have. Write about wishes you hope for, and dates you want to do with them. Write about the movie you watched tonight and things that are going on in your life. This journal will be a special gift to give your dom when you finally come together.

Task #8: Complete Your Night Time Routine

- Drink 1 glass of water
- Brush your teeth
- Turn off all social media and computers. Power down for the night.
- Pull on fresh pajamas
- If you have a picture book, (or checked one out from the library), lay down in bed and quietly read your book. If you don't have a picture book, listen to a read aloud picture book on YouTube. (There are bunches of videos!)
- Reduce your room lighting to a simple side lamp or fairy lights. Quiet the mind.
- Turn on soft lullaby music or classical music on YouTube

As you begin to feel groggy, turn everything off, snuggle up to your plushie and drift off to sleep. (Make sure to get those 7–8 hours of rest in!).

Day 15: Discovering New Sensations

Welcome to Day 15 of your Little Training! Today is all about discovering new tactile sensations to enhance your time in little space. If you walk down any children's toy area, you'll notice that most toys have some tactile design involved. A plushie has furry hair. A toy can squeak or make a rattling sound. Toys are designed to captivate and draw in your senses. As a Little you can be selective to discover which types of sensations you most enjoy while in Little space, then incorporate items accordingly. For example: if you know that you prefer snuggles in Little space often, try using an electric heating blanket to rest under while in Little space. The gentle heat can soothe you into deeper relaxation as you watch a kid show. Other Littles love the feeling of having a pacifier in their mouth. They love to look at themselves in the mirror and visually see a binky there along with having the pacifier rest on their tongue.

Still other Littles prefer swaddling up in blankets, or what I affectionately call "becoming a burrito". Have you ever wondered why it feels so natural to wrap up in a blanket when we're sick, or having a bad day? As an infant, we are swaddled almost immediately from when we enter the world. Over the first year of our life, swaddling from head to toe is a sensation that gives comfort to our systems. This feeling lies dormant as we age, but being a Little you can tap into that feeling of security and comfort as you wrap up in a giant, soft blanket in Little space.

Take advantage of playing around with textures and sensations. Give bottle-feeding a try and see if it brings up emotion in your belly. Run your fingertips over various fabrics at a cloth store and find out if you enjoy faux fur, leather, silk, etc. Understanding what patterns, textures, and sensations you enjoy will help deepen and enhance your Little play space.

Today's Challenge: Choose one new sensation or item that stimulates your senses and use it in Little Space. Record your feelings in your evening journal letter.

After you have completed your challenge, please move on to your day 15 tasks.

Day 15 Tasks:

Task #1: Complete Your Morning Routine
- Drink 1 glass of water as soon as you wake up
- Wash your face
- Brush your teeth
- Throw your shower towel into the dryer (if available) and have it tumbling on low-medium heat while you hop into the shower.
- Shower up. While in the shower, think of a song you used to love as a child. Sing that song to yourself as you lather up. Then wrap yourself up in your warm towel afterward. Ahhh...
- Take time to pick out an outfit that is both comfortable, yet makes you feel pretty.

- Put on sunscreen and Chapstick
- Lotion your skin with baby lotion

Task #2: Meditate for 15 minutes

If you have a phone, I want you to download the FREE app. Headspace. It has guided meditation apps that are picked by the program based upon your current mood. If you do not have a phone, go onto YouTube and follow a 15-minute guided meditation video. Allow your breathing to calm and relax your body. Let go of your stresses and fears. Simply be. This daily practice is designed to train you to build up patience in sitting still as you will need to do for your dominant in the future.

Task #3: Browse DDLG/LB Fashion Online

Begin browsing fashion online to formulate your own unique little style! You can also see previous chapters (III., IV., and V. in this book for product and clothing suggestions). There is a style for everyone. Go and find yours!

Task #4: Time to start your normal day, but don't forget your Little snacks!

Whether you're going to school, or staying at home, as you're doing your normal daily schedule I want you to take several breaks throughout the day to refuel with a glass of water and a small snack. These snacks should specifically remind you of Little Me. Some suggestions include: goldfish crackers, animal crackers, cheese cubes, lunchables, cheerios, etc.

Task #5: Stretch those muscles for 20 minutes of exercise!

This act of self-care will keep you feeling good and your body strong. Pick an activity that you already enjoy doing and exercise for 20 minutes.

Task #6: Evening D/s Movie

Every day for the next 25 days I want you to watch a movie that I've hand-picked that is designed to make you think about qualities that dominants should have. Characters in these movies all portray traits that most dom's exude. Think about the relationship dynamics and then follow up in Task #6 with your evening journal reflection letter.

Tonight's D/s Movie is: *Leap Year (2010)*

Task #7: Evening Journal Reflection

Now that your day is starting to wind down and you have completed your first D/s movie, I want you to do an evening journal reflection. Instead of a typical diary entry, I want you to write a letter to your future dominant. You can begin by saying: Dear Future Dom... or Dear Dominant... or Dear Daddy/Mommy.... write what feels natural to you. Think about the qualities you want your dominant to have. Write about wishes you hope for, and dates you want to do with them. Write about the movie you watched tonight and things that are going on in your life. This journal will be a special gift to give your dom when you finally come together.

Task #8: Complete Your Night Time Routine

- Drink 1 glass of water
- Brush your teeth
- Turn off all social media and computers. Power down for the night.
- Pull on fresh pajamas
- If you have a picture book, (or checked one out from the library), lay down in bed and quietly read your book. If you don't have a picture book, listen to a read aloud picture book on YouTube. (There are bunches of videos!)
- Reduce your room lighting to a simple side lamp or fairy lights. Quiet the mind.
- Turn on soft lullaby music or classical music on YouTube

As you begin to feel groggy, turn everything off, snuggle up to your plushie and drift off to sleep. (Make sure to get those 7-8 hours of rest in!).

Day 16: Creating a Little Vision Board

I firmly believe in the power of dreaming and daydreaming. It is healthy for the mind to dream, hope, believe, and feel inspired. Just as you plan goals for your everyday life, so too, should you plan goals and dream big for your little space! Today's task will focus on you creating a dream vision board to keep somewhere in your room. You can use poster-board or cardboard, whatever you have on hand. There is no size requirement. I just want you become inspired to be the Little that you wish to be. Pinterest and Google Images has a host of DDLG/LB images for you to draw inspiration from as you put together a collage of words and images that resonate with you. Think about what type of Little you wish to be. What type of dominant do you hope to find? Is there a fantasy in your mind that you wish to act out?

Many Littles love playing around with various fashion styles. Some Littles dive head first into Lolita fashion, while others prefer a more edgy punk-rock, yet kawaii style. Get creative with your vision board. Whip out the glitter and gel markers and let your imagination run wild. Write words on your board that inspires you in Little space. Having a visual reminder of where you want to go as a submissive and Little will help you to articulate your feelings and dreams to your future dominant.

Today's Challenge: Search the internet, magazines, toy catalogs, etc. for images that resonate with you as a Little. Then cut and paste them together into a collage to create a vision board. Get as creative as you'd like!

After you've completed your Little vision board, please move on to complete your day 16 tasks.

Day 16 Tasks:

Task #1: Complete Your Morning Routine
- Drink 1 glass of water as soon as you wake up
- Wash your face
- Brush your teeth
- Throw your shower towel into the dryer (if available) and have it tumbling on low-medium heat while you hop into the shower.
- Shower up. While in the shower, think of a song you used to love as a child. Sing that song to yourself as you lather up. Then wrap yourself up in your warm towel afterward. Ahhh...
- Take time to pick out an outfit that is both comfortable, yet makes you feel pretty.
- Put on sunscreen and Chapstick
- Lotion your skin with baby lotion

Task #2: Meditate for 15 minutes
If you have a phone, I want you to download the FREE app. Headspace. It has guided meditation apps that are picked by the program based upon your current mood. If you do not have a phone, go onto

YouTube and follow a 15-minute guided meditation video. Allow your breathing to calm and relax your body. Let go of your stresses and fears. Simply be. This daily practice is designed to train you to build up patience in sitting still as you will need to do for your dominant in the future.

Task #3: Browse DDLG/LB Fashion Online

Begin browsing fashion online to formulate your own unique little style! You can also see previous chapters (III., IV., and V. in this book for product and clothing suggestions). There is a style for everyone. Go and find yours!

Task #4: Time to start your normal day, but don't forget your Little snacks!

Whether you're going to school, or staying at home, as you're doing your normal daily schedule I want you to take several breaks throughout the day to refuel with a glass of water and a small snack. These snacks should specifically remind you of Little Me. Some suggestions include: goldfish crackers, animal crackers, cheese cubes, lunchables, cheerios, etc.

Task #5: Stretch those muscles for 20 minutes of exercise!

This act of self-care will keep you feeling good and your body strong. Pick an activity that you already enjoy doing and exercise for 20 minutes.

Task #6: Evening D/s Movie

Every day for the next 25 days I want you to watch a movie that I've hand-picked that is designed to make you think about qualities that dominants should have. Characters in these movies all portray traits that most dom's exude. Think about the relationship dynamics and then follow up in Task #6 with your evening journal reflection letter.

Tonight's D/s Movie is: *Frozen (2013)*

Task #7: Evening Journal Reflection

Now that your day is starting to wind down and you have completed your first D/s movie, I want you to do an evening journal reflection. Instead of a typical diary entry, I want you to write a letter to your future dominant. You can begin by saying: Dear Future Dom... or Dear Dominant... or Dear Daddy/Mommy.... write what feels natural to you. Think about the qualities you want your dominant to have. Write about wishes you hope for, and dates you want to do with them. Write about the movie you watched tonight and things that are going on in your life. This journal will be a special gift to give your dom when you finally come together.

Task #8: Complete Your Night Time Routine

- Drink 1 glass of water
- Brush your teeth
- Turn off all social media and computers. Power down for the night.
- Pull on fresh pajamas

- If you have a picture book, (or checked one out from the library), lay down in bed and quietly read your book. If you don't have a picture book, listen to a read aloud picture book on YouTube. (There are bunches of videos!)
- Reduce your room lighting to a simple side lamp or fairy lights. Quiet the mind.
- Turn on soft lullaby music or classical music on YouTube

As you begin to feel groggy, turn everything off, snuggle up to your plushie and drift off to sleep. (Make sure to get those 7-8 hours of rest in!).

Day 17: Connecting With Others

Welcome to Day 17 of your Little Training! As we grow near the completion of your 25-day training, we will start to take the proverbial training wheels off of you, so that you feel confident taking off on your own. Today's focus is an optional task of connecting with other Littles. While the subject of DDLG/LB can be taboo in some circles, there are literally thousands of Littles out there who are "loud and proud" in their identity. Learning to connect with other Littles online is an excellent way to continue feeling Little while being solo. There are plenty of forums online for you to use a forum tag/ fake name to talk to others. By talking to other Littles, you can continue to learn and grow as you "play" with others.

Below are some forum sites specifically for little girls and boys to help you connect more with the community:
- **DDLG Friends** https://www.ddlgfriends.com/
- **DDLG Forum** https://www.ddlgforum.com/
- **LittleSpace Online** https://www.littlespaceonline.com/
- **ADISC AB/ DL/ IC Support Community** https://www.adisc.org/forum/index.php
- **FetLife** https://fetlife.com/

There are also voice servers online in which you can use a headset and microphone to verbally talk to other Littles and Dominants. One such server is:
- **DDLG Forum on Discord** https://www.discordlist.me/servers/454703542788292618

Talking to strangers and new Littles online can seem like a daunting task, especially if you've never spoken to anyone online before. But, if you choose to connect online you will quickly learn why it's such a popular way to socialize. Since you aren't face to face, you can be dressed however you like and the only thing people will see are the things you type, or listen to the sound of your voice. There is *a lot* less pressure to look a certain way or act in a certain manner. If you're too nervous to chat, then I encourage you to visit these sites and just browse the forums. Read what other Littles and Dom's have posted. Get a feel for what people in the community are talking about. Maybe you'll learn something new as you sift through the forum threads!

Today's Optional Challenge: Pick one of the online forum sites listed above and create a username and password (pick a forum name!). Then find a welcome thread and say hello to everyone. You can post that you're new to the Little lifestyle and you welcome any advice and feedback. Then sit back and see who replies!

When you've completed your challenge for the day, please move to complete your day 17 tasks.

Day 17 Tasks:

Task #1: Complete Your Morning Routine

- Drink 1 glass of water as soon as you wake up
- Wash your face
- Brush your teeth
- Throw your shower towel into the dryer (if available) and have it tumbling on low-medium heat while you hop into the shower.
- Shower up. While in the shower, think of a song you used to love as a child. Sing that song to yourself as you lather up. Then wrap yourself up in your warm towel afterward. Ahhh...
- Take time to pick out an outfit that is both comfortable, yet makes you feel pretty.
- Put on sunscreen and Chapstick
- Lotion your skin with baby lotion

Task #2: Meditate for 15 minutes

If you have a phone, I want you to download the FREE app. Headspace. It has guided meditation apps that are picked by the program based upon your current mood. If you do not have a phone, go onto YouTube and follow a 15-minute guided meditation video. Allow your breathing to calm and relax your body. Let go of your stresses and fears. Simply be. This daily practice is designed to train you to build up patience in sitting still as you will need to do for your dominant in the future.

Task #3: Browse DDLG/LB Fashion Online

Begin browsing fashion online to formulate your own unique little style! You can also see previous chapters (III., IV., and V. in this book for product and clothing suggestions). There is a style for everyone. Go and find yours!

Task #4: Time to start your normal day, but don't forget your Little snacks!

Whether you're going to school, or staying at home, as you're doing your normal daily schedule I want you to take several breaks throughout the day to refuel with a glass of water and a small snack. These snacks should specifically remind you of Little Me. Some suggestions include: goldfish crackers, animal crackers, cheese cubes, lunchables, cheerios, etc.

Task #5: Stretch those muscles for 20 minutes of exercise!

This act of self-care will keep you feeling good and your body strong. Pick an activity that you already enjoy doing and exercise for 20 minutes.

Task #6: Evening D/s Movie

Every day for the next 25 days I want you to watch a movie that I've hand-picked that is designed to make you think about qualities that dominants should have. Characters in these movies all portray

traits that most dom's exude. Think about the relationship dynamics and then follow up in Task #6 with your evening journal reflection letter.

Tonight's D/s Movie is: *Just You (2013), a Taiwanese Romantic-Comedy TV show with strong D/s themes.*

Task #7: Evening Journal Reflection

Now that your day is starting to wind down and you have completed your first D/s movie, I want you to do an evening journal reflection. Instead of a typical diary entry, I want you to write a letter to your future dominant. You can begin by saying: Dear Future Dom... or Dear Dominant... or Dear Daddy/Mommy.... write what feels natural to you. Think about the qualities you want your dominant to have. Write about wishes you hope for, and dates you want to do with them. Write about the movie you watched tonight and things that are going on in your life. This journal will be a special gift to give your dom when you finally come together.

Task #8: Complete Your Night Time Routine

- Drink 1 glass of water
- Brush your teeth
- Turn off all social media and computers. Power down for the night.
- Pull on fresh pajamas
- If you have a picture book, (or checked one out from the library), lay down in bed and quietly read your book. If you don't have a picture book, listen to a read aloud picture book on YouTube. (There are bunches of videos!)
- Reduce your room lighting to a simple side lamp or fairy lights. Quiet the mind.
- Turn on soft lullaby music or classical music on YouTube

As you begin to feel groggy, turn everything off, snuggle up to your plushie and drift off to sleep. (Make sure to get those 7-8 hours of rest in!).

Day 18: Drawing Confidence From Role Models in the Community

Welcome to Day 18 of your Little Training! Today we will examine a few people who are not necessarily Littles in our community, but they can be inspirational nonetheless. My wish for you is that by seeing others who have pave their own way (through fashion, music, a BDSM lifestyle, etc.) you will gain more confidence in being your own authentic self. The ultimate goal is for you to feel a strong sense of self in what you like and enjoy. That way, you will be able to move forward with ease as you continue to get more involved in the community and connect with others.

Here are a few individuals who have dedicated their life to being different and marching proudly to their own beat:

1. **Rihanna:** Take a look at Rihanna's music and it's no shocker that this A-list musician/celebrity is into BDSM. In her music videos "Disturbia", "S&M", and "Rude Boy" she flaunts her feminism and sexuality with risque outfits and shows off images of submissives in bondage.

2. **Dita Von Teese:** If you've never watched a burlesque show before, I encourage you to watch the movie, "Moulin Rouge" (2001). Dita Von Teese helped repopularize the burlesque movement which involves dancers in risque outfits teasing the senses of their audience without being so forward like that of a strip club. It's art and dance, with partial nudity. You can draw inspiration of how to wear lingerie in a sexy way by clicking through her Instagram page.

3. **Pixielocks:** Attention all kawaii fans. If you're into Lolita fashion, rainbows, unicorns, anime, and cosplay, this next person is just for you! Pixielocks (aka Jillian Vessey) is a Canadian Youtuber who has dedicated her life towards pushing kawaii fashion. Check out her Instagram and YouTube channel to bask in all things pastel and happy.

4. **Julia Zelg:** This goth-kawaii Youtuber has her own music out, gives makeup tutorials, and has plenty of videos for you to draw inspiration from if you're excited to dabble in a more edgy little fashion style.

5. **Binkie Princess:** Binkie Princess is a controversial DDLG Youtuber, but you have to applaud her because she has paved the way for the community in terms of putting DDLG in the spotlight. She has taken much criticism for her videos, but there is a strong resilience in this little ABDL! Her passion to continue to make content, connect with her daddy in a separate channel, and push forward despite thousands of people giving her negative comments is truly commendable.

6. **Little Moo Moo:** Little Moo Moo is a more wholesome DDLG Youtuber who is a ray of sunshine on her channel. She loves to focus on unboxing videos, music, and just chatting on live stream. Her videos feel very warm and personal as she connects with her audience. If you're looking for a great role model and inspiration as you begin your path as a Little, look no further.

Today's Challenge: In your evening journal reflection, write about one of these role models that inspires you in your journey as a Little. (Or pick another one of your own!). Reflect on what you like about them and how it makes you feel.

When you've completed today's challenge, please move on to complete your day 18 tasks.

Day 18 Tasks:

Task #1: Complete Your Morning Routine
- Drink 1 glass of water as soon as you wake up
- Wash your face
- Brush your teeth
- Throw your shower towel into the dryer (if available) and have it tumbling on low-medium heat while you hop into the shower.
- Shower up. While in the shower, think of a song you used to love as a child. Sing that song to yourself as you lather up. Then wrap yourself up in your warm towel afterward. Ahhh...
- Take time to pick out an outfit that is both comfortable, yet makes you feel pretty.
- Put on sunscreen and Chapstick
- Lotion your skin with baby lotion

Task #2: Meditate for 15 minutes
If you have a phone, I want you to download the FREE app. Headspace. It has guided meditation apps that are picked by the program based upon your current mood. If you do not have a phone, go onto YouTube and follow a 15-minute guided meditation video. Allow your breathing to calm and relax your body. Let go of your stresses and fears. Simply be. This daily practice is designed to train you to build up patience in sitting still as you will need to do for your dominant in the future.

Task #3: Browse DDLG/LB Fashion Online
Begin browsing fashion online to formulate your own unique little style! You can also see previous chapters (III., IV., and V. in this book for product and clothing suggestions). There is a style for everyone. Go and find yours!

Task #4: Time to start your normal day, but don't forget your Little snacks!
Whether you're going to school, or staying at home, as you're doing your normal daily schedule I want you to take several breaks throughout the day to refuel with a glass of water and a small snack. These snacks should specifically remind you of Little Me. Some suggestions include: goldfish crackers, animal crackers, cheese cubes, lunchables, cheerios, etc.

Task #5: Stretch those muscles for 20 minutes of exercise!
This act of self-care will keep you feeling good and your body strong. Pick an activity that you already enjoy doing and exercise for 20 minutes.

Task #6: Evening D/s Movie

Every day for the next 25 days I want you to watch a movie that I've hand-picked that is designed to make you think about qualities that dominants should have. Characters in these movies all portray traits that most dom's exude. Think about the relationship dynamics and then follow up in Task #6 with your evening journal reflection letter.

Tonight's D/s Movie is: *Pirate's Passage (2015)*

Task #7: Evening Journal Reflection

Now that your day is starting to wind down and you have completed your first D/s movie, I want you to do an evening journal reflection. Instead of a typical diary entry, I want you to write a letter to your future dominant. You can begin by saying: Dear Future Dom... or Dear Dominant... or Dear Daddy/Mommy.... write what feels natural to you. Think about the qualities you want your dominant to have. Write about wishes you hope for, and dates you want to do with them. Write about the movie you watched tonight and things that are going on in your life. This journal will be a special gift to give your dom when you finally come together.

Task #8: Complete Your Night Time Routine

- Drink 1 glass of water
- Brush your teeth
- Turn off all social media and computers. Power down for the night.
- Pull on fresh pajamas
- If you have a picture book, (or checked one out from the library), lay down in bed and quietly read your book. If you don't have a picture book, listen to a read aloud picture book on YouTube. (There are bunches of videos!)
- Reduce your room lighting to a simple side lamp or fairy lights. Quiet the mind.
- Turn on soft lullaby music or classical music on YouTube

As you begin to feel groggy, turn everything off, snuggle up to your plushie and drift off to sleep. (Make sure to get those 7-8 hours of rest in!).

Day 19: Submission in Modern History

Welcome to Day 19 of your Little Training! Today's focus will be examining submission throughout cultures across the world. The word submission has long carried a negative connotation attached to it. This is especially true since the rise of global feminism began in the late 1960's. While some might view women who voluntarily submit as "weak" or "lesser than", this couldn't be farther from the truth. True submission comes from a place of love rather than fear. This is the same in a D/s relationship. The Dominant/Master/Partner must guide with a loving and understanding hand to gain the submissives trust. If the two parties cannot create a symbiotic relationship built on trust, love, and understanding, then the bond is doomed to fail. Submission is not the relinquishment of an opinion, but rather the surrender of trust unto the dominant.

Throughout history leading to the present submission has been a major part of cultures across the globe. Let's take a look at a few examples:

- Biblical submission within Christianity has led to widespread submission in many countries across the globe. This form of submission originated from the Bible verse in Ephesians 5:21-25 in which women are called to submit unto their husbands.
- In Islam, there is a major misconception that women are submissive to their husbands. While the Quran clearly states that men and women are viewed as equal, it also dictates that women should refrain from showing skin except to their husbands. This form of submission can be found in the Quran, 24:30-31.
- In Japanese culture, Geishas are not submissive to the patrons that they perform for. However, these women do obey the women that own the geisha houses and train them.
- In African culture, many countries are influenced by Christianity and follow the form of Biblical submission where a woman is expected to serve her husband fully and take care of the home.
- In Filipino culture, women are raised from a very early age to learn respect, good manners, and understanding so that as they grow up they can become good mothers and submissive wives.
- In Korean culture, although most women enter the workforce it is expected that upon marriage and the arrival of the first child, the woman will give up her career and stay home to raise the baby.
- In Chinese culture, while modern day China does have equal gender laws, there are many regions within China that treat men with superiority than women.
- In Indian culture there is a large amount of societal pressure for females to be raised to be submissive to their husbands and in-laws. Many marriages are pre-arranged and divided by socio-economic status as well as religion. This dictates who marries who and usually the females end up living with their husband and in-laws to help care for the home and their children.

So, if females in particular have been forced into submission over the course of centuries, why then, would anyone *voluntarily* choose to become a slave, Little, pet, or kajira? How is cultural submission different from the BDSM community? For starters, in a D/s relationship both parties are adults who enter into the bond consensually. Nothing is forced, and nothing is pressured to make happen. Instead it is the connection of two souls, one who yearns to nurture and care for the submissive, and the other who longs to please their dominant and make them smile. It is a relationship bred of love and trust. In many ways, it is the deepest type of relationship one can have, because it takes so much work! However, it is incredibly rewarding when both parties trust each other completely and feel satisfied.

Today's Challenge: For your challenge today, I want you to reflect on why you want to become a submissive to a dominant. Being a Little is one form of submission, but it is submission nonetheless. Why do you want to submit to your dominant? How does the thought of submitting make you feel? Write your thoughts down in your evening journal letter.

After you've completed today's challenge, please move on to complete your day 19 tasks.

Day 19 Tasks:

Task #1: Complete Your Morning Routine
- Drink 1 glass of water as soon as you wake up
- Wash your face
- Brush your teeth
- Throw your shower towel into the dryer (if available) and have it tumbling on low-medium heat while you hop into the shower.
- Shower up. While in the shower, think of a song you used to love as a child. Sing that song to yourself as you lather up. Then wrap yourself up in your warm towel afterward. Ahhh...
- Take time to pick out an outfit that is both comfortable, yet makes you feel pretty.
- Put on sunscreen and Chapstick
- Lotion your skin with baby lotion

Task #2: Meditate for 15 minutes
If you have a phone, I want you to download the FREE app. Headspace. It has guided meditation apps that are picked by the program based upon your current mood. If you do not have a phone, go onto YouTube and follow a 15-minute guided meditation video. Allow your breathing to calm and relax your body. Let go of your stresses and fears. Simply be. This daily practice is designed to train you to build up patience in sitting still as you will need to do for your dominant in the future.

Task #3: Browse DDLG/LB Fashion Online
Begin browsing fashion online to formulate your own unique little style! You can also see previous chapters (III., IV., and V. in this book for product and clothing suggestions). There is a style for everyone. Go and find yours!

Task #4: Time to start your normal day, but don't forget your Little snacks!

Whether you're going to school, or staying at home, as you're doing your normal daily schedule I want you to take several breaks throughout the day to refuel with a glass of water and a small snack. These snacks should specifically remind you of Little Me. Some suggestions include: goldfish crackers, animal crackers, cheese cubes, lunchables, cheerios, etc.

Task #5: Stretch those muscles for 20 minutes of exercise!

This act of self-care will keep you feeling good and your body strong. Pick an activity that you already enjoy doing and exercise for 20 minutes.

Task #6: Evening D/s Movie

Every day for the next 25 days I want you to watch a movie that I've hand-picked that is designed to make you think about qualities that dominants should have. Characters in these movies all portray traits that most dom's exude. Think about the relationship dynamics and then follow up in Task #6 with your evening journal reflection letter.

Tonight's D/s Movie is: *Rodeo & Juliet (2015)*

Task #7: Evening Journal Reflection

Now that your day is starting to wind down and you have completed your first D/s movie, I want you to do an evening journal reflection. Instead of a typical diary entry, I want you to write a letter to your future dominant. You can begin by saying: Dear Future Dom... or Dear Dominant... or Dear Daddy/Mommy.... write what feels natural to you. Think about the qualities you want your dominant to have. Write about wishes you hope for, and dates you want to do with them. Write about the movie you watched tonight and things that are going on in your life. This journal will be a special gift to give your dom when you finally come together.

Task #8: Complete Your Night Time Routine

- Drink 1 glass of water
- Brush your teeth
- Turn off all social media and computers. Power down for the night.
- Pull on fresh pajamas
- If you have a picture book, (or checked one out from the library), lay down in bed and quietly read your book. If you don't have a picture book, listen to a read aloud picture book on YouTube. (There are bunches of videos!)
- Reduce your room lighting to a simple side lamp or fairy lights. Quiet the mind.
- Turn on soft lullaby music or classical music on YouTube

As you begin to feel groggy, turn everything off, snuggle up to your plushie and drift off to sleep. (Make sure to get those 7-8 hours of rest in!).

Day 20: Learning About Other Submissive Styles

Welcome to Day 20 of your Little Training! As you're diving more into the lifestyle and community you will quickly learn that no two Littles are alike and the tastes that each Little has varies. Some Littles will tell you that they are part-Little and part-something else. This is because being a Little is a form of submission. There are various types of submission and labels within the DDLG/LB community that people identify with. So, let's begin to examine each of the major labels. There might be more out there than listed here. My apologies if I forgot any! Now let's dive in together.

Within the D/l community some major labels include:
- Littles
- Middles
- Baby Girls
- Lolitas (A fashion style that accentuates the sweet innocence of youth/ looks like a baby doll)
- Little Sissies (A boy or man who enjoys wearing little clothing)
- Bubbies (An affectionate term for someone you love)
- Age Players (a person who roleplays as a little)
- Age Regressors
- Sexual littles
- Non-sexual littles
- Caregivers
- Mommys
- Daddys
- Aunties
- Babysitters
- Big Brothers
- Big Sisters

Some other forms of submission within the BDSM community that littles might adopt behaviors, traits, etc. of include:

1. **Kinkster:** is someone who practices various kinks usually within the privacy of the bedroom. They generally do not live their kink on a full-time basis, but prefer to keep their kink lifestyle and their normal lifestyle separate.

2. **A Taken in Hand Relationship:** Usually revolves around Christian Biblical submission where the dominant (usually a man) is the head of the household. The submissives duties are usually domestic related, to care for the home, cook, etc. The dominant rules with a stern hand.

3. **Dominance/Submissive (D/s):** is the main branch of BDSM where there is a dominant who can be a Master and the submissive is theirs completely. The sub relinquishes total

power to the dominant. In return, the dominant cares for the sub with everything they have. This can be on a part or full-time basis and a contract is always agreed upon first.

4. **A Switch:** A person engaged in a D/s relationship that is fluid where they are sometimes the dominant and sometimes the submissive. A switch usually partners with another switch.

5. **Consensual Slavery:** A submissive who voluntarily surrenders total control of their life to their dominant. There is usually no "off" time. The slave lives full-time as a slave to help care for their Master. Punishment is usually corporal. An example of this can be seen in Gorean subculture, called a kajira.

6. **A Pet:** is a submissive that acts and is treated like a pet by their Master. They can be taken for walks, eat from a bowl on the floor, and wear tools and outfits to enhance their pet play.

7. **Code d' Odalisque (Pleasure Slave):** is a submissive that is usually kept naked 24/7 with the exception of wearing a collar at all times. They are never punished with physical punishments because the Master usually wants to keep their body pristine. The pleasure slave is expected to be sexually ready for their Master at all times.

8. **Masochist:** a submissive that derives pleasure and climax through physical pain. The sadist is a dominant that derives pleasure and climax through inflicting control and pain over their masochist. This is usually achieved through bondage, whipping, spanking, etc.

Today's Challenge: Reflect on the various types of paths to submission and see if there are any other forms of submission that interest you. If there are, write about them in your evening journal reflection. If not, that's fine too. Write about how you feel about the other forms of submission. Was there a path that completely turned you off? If so, why?

After you have completed today's challenge, please move on to complete your day 20 tasks.

Day 20 Tasks:

Task #1: Complete Your Morning Routine
- Drink 1 glass of water as soon as you wake up
- Wash your face
- Brush your teeth
- Throw your shower towel into the dryer (if available) and have it tumbling on low-medium heat while you hop into the shower.
- Shower up. While in the shower, think of a song you used to love as a child. Sing that song to yourself as you lather up. Then wrap yourself up in your warm towel afterward. Ahhh...
- Take time to pick out an outfit that is both comfortable, yet makes you feel pretty.
- Put on sunscreen and Chapstick
- Lotion your skin with baby lotion

Task #2: Meditate for 15 minutes

If you have a phone, I want you to download the FREE app. Headspace. It has guided meditation apps that are picked by the program based upon your current mood. If you do not have a phone, go onto YouTube and follow a 15-minute guided meditation video. Allow your breathing to calm and relax your body. Let go of your stresses and fears. Simply be. This daily practice is designed to train you to build up patience in sitting still as you will need to do for your dominant in the future.

Task #3: Browse DDLG/LB Fashion Online

Begin browsing fashion online to formulate your own unique little style! You can also see previous chapters (III., IV., and V. in this book for product and clothing suggestions). There is a style for everyone. Go and find yours!

Task #4: Time to start your normal day, but don't forget your Little snacks!

Whether you're going to school, or staying at home, as you're doing your normal daily schedule I want you to take several breaks throughout the day to refuel with a glass of water and a small snack. These snacks should specifically remind you of Little Me. Some suggestions include: goldfish crackers, animal crackers, cheese cubes, lunchables, cheerios, etc.

Task #5: Stretch those muscles for 20 minutes of exercise!

This act of self-care will keep you feeling good and your body strong. Pick an activity that you already enjoy doing and exercise for 20 minutes.

Task #6: Evening D/s Movie

Every day for the next 25 days I want you to watch a movie that I've hand-picked that is designed to make you think about qualities that dominants should have. Characters in these movies all portray traits that most dom's exude. Think about the relationship dynamics and then follow up in Task #6 with your evening journal reflection letter.

Tonight's D/s Movie is: *Two Weeks Notice (2002)*

Task #7: Evening Journal Reflection

Now that your day is starting to wind down and you have completed your first D/s movie, I want you to do an evening journal reflection. Instead of a typical diary entry, I want you to write a letter to your future dominant. You can begin by saying: Dear Future Dom... or Dear Dominant... or Dear Daddy/Mommy.... write what feels natural to you. Think about the qualities you want your dominant to have. Write about wishes you hope for, and dates you want to do with them. Write about the movie you watched tonight and things that are going on in your life. This journal will be a special gift to give your dom when you finally come together.

Task #8: Complete Your Night Time Routine
- Drink 1 glass of water

- Brush your teeth
- Turn off all social media and computers. Power down for the night.
- Pull on fresh pajamas
- If you have a picture book, (or checked one out from the library), lay down in bed and quietly read your book. If you don't have a picture book, listen to a read aloud picture book on YouTube. (There are bunches of videos!)
- Reduce your room lighting to a simple side lamp or fairy lights. Quiet the mind.
- Turn on soft lullaby music or classical music on YouTube

As you begin to feel groggy, turn everything off, snuggle up to your plushie and drift off to sleep. (Make sure to get those 7-8 hours of rest in!).

Day 21: Video Games For Solo Littles

Welcome to Day 21 of your Little Training! If you haven't noticed by now, I am a giant nerd, and my daddy is too. As such, this training wouldn't be complete without showing you how DDLG/LB has influenced even the video game market. As a solo little there are many games available on the market for you to play to keep you feeling little while you are on your own. Let's begin by breaking these games into two main categories: Single player games and Multiplayer games

Single player games are design for you to engage with the program to achieve a certain outcome. If you've never gone to the platform, Steam, it is a free video game hosting platform. You register for free, then you will have access to thousands of games to download – some for purchase and some for free. One specific type of single player game is called a visual novel. Like a choose your own adventure book, these games are formatted for you to determine the outcome of the story as you make decisions throughout the course of the game. These games can be especially beneficial for a solo Little because it allows you to role-play and connect with the characters in the game while controlling the fate of the story line. Some excellent single player games that I recommend include:
- The Men of Yoshiwara
- Dream Daddy
- Coming Out on Top
- Nekopara vol. 1
- Amorous
- Trick and Treat
- Tokyo School Life
- Montaro

Multiplayer games have long been an attraction for people within the BDSM community because these games allow the formation of guilds. MMORPG or a Massively Multiplayer Online Role-Playing Game, allows you to explore within a vast universe with other players from all over the world. By creating an avatar that you design, you are able to explore and adventure beyond the typical hack and slash format. These games cater to the D/s community because you can create BDSM events, night clubs, have private guild halls, and more. Some of the more well-known MMORPG that have a thriving BDSM player base include:
- **World of Warcraft:** This MMO is over 10 years old and has a player population of over a million players. The primary servers for connecting with other role-players include: Wyrmrest Accord, Moon Guard, and Emerald Dream. World of Warcraft has a $14.99 per month subscription in addition to purchasing the game off of the Blizzard website. There are dozens of RP guilds and BDSM themed guilds, as well as brothels, and kink-specific guilds. Check out the specific server forums on recruiting guilds.
- **Final Fantasy XIV:** This subscription-based game also costs $14.99 per month plus the cost of the game from Square Enix. Players interested in connecting with BDSM guilds, should

aim to roll a character on the servers: Leviathan or Balmung. This fantasy-based game can cater to your kitten fantasies as one of the main races are the cat humanoids Miqo'te.

- **Guild Wars 2:** This is an MMO that does not have a subscription fee but requires purchase of the base game and any other expansions you desire to unlock content. Players interested in role-player should aim for the servers: Tarnished Coast (US) or Piken Square (EU). It has a very good character customization feature and an extensive wardrobe system and so you can play dress up to your heart's content.
- **Second Life:** This MMO allows players to create the world in which you play. By purchasing laurels, the in-game currency, you can build a home, customize your avatar and so much more. A major appeal of this game is that players can convert in game currency to real money. Many players establish businesses within the game as a secondary source of income. There are many servers within the Second Life world that cater to the BDSM community with nightclubs, events, hotels, etc.
- **Lord of the Rings Online:** This MMO has a thriving RP community on the servers Laurelin (EU) and Landroval (US) because of their unique armor customization as well as the rich lore and the beauty of the world developed by the game designers. If you've ever fantasized about wanting to be part of Tolkien's world, then this game is perfect for you.

Today's Challenge: Choose one of the games listed above and research it. Find a game that resonates with you and give it a try. Then, reflect on your experience in your evening journal letter.

After you complete today's challenge, please complete your day 21 tasks.

Day 21 Tasks:

Task #1: Complete Your Morning Routine
- Drink 1 glass of water as soon as you wake up
- Wash your face
- Brush your teeth
- Throw your shower towel into the dryer (if available) and have it tumbling on low-medium heat while you hop into the shower.
- Shower up. While in the shower, think of a song you used to love as a child. Sing that song to yourself as you lather up. Then wrap yourself up in your warm towel afterward. Ahhh...
- Take time to pick out an outfit that is both comfortable, yet makes you feel pretty.
- Put on sunscreen and Chapstick
- Lotion your skin with baby lotion

Task #2: Meditate for 15 minutes
If you have a phone, I want you to download the FREE app. Headspace. It has guided meditation apps that are picked by the program based upon your current mood. If you do not have a phone, go onto YouTube and follow a 15-minute guided meditation video. Allow your breathing to calm and relax your

body. Let go of your stresses and fears. Simply be. This daily practice is designed to train you to build up patience in sitting still as you will need to do for your dominant in the future.

Task #3: Browse DDLG/LB Fashion Online

Begin browsing fashion online to formulate your own unique little style! You can also see previous chapters (III., IV., and V. in this book for product and clothing suggestions). There is a style for everyone. Go and find yours!

Task #4: Time to start your normal day, but don't forget your Little snacks!

Whether you're going to school, or staying at home, as you're doing your normal daily schedule I want you to take several breaks throughout the day to refuel with a glass of water and a small snack. These snacks should specifically remind you of Little Me. Some suggestions include: goldfish crackers, animal crackers, cheese cubes, lunchables, cheerios, etc.

Task #5: Stretch those muscles for 20 minutes of exercise!

This act of self-care will keep you feeling good and your body strong. Pick an activity that you already enjoy doing and exercise for 20 minutes.

Task #6: Evening D/s Movie

Every day for the next 25 days I want you to watch a movie that I've hand-picked that is designed to make you think about qualities that dominants should have. Characters in these movies all portray traits that most dom's exude. Think about the relationship dynamics and then follow up in Task #6 with your evening journal reflection letter.

Tonight's D/s Movie is: *An Education (2009)*

Task #7: Evening Journal Reflection

Now that your day is starting to wind down and you have completed your first D/s movie, I want you to do an evening journal reflection. Instead of a typical diary entry, I want you to write a letter to your future dominant. You can begin by saying: Dear Future Dom... or Dear Dominant... or Dear Daddy/Mommy.... write what feels natural to you. Think about the qualities you want your dominant to have. Write about wishes you hope for, and dates you want to do with them. Write about the movie you watched tonight and things that are going on in your life. This journal will be a special gift to give your dom when you finally come together.

Task #8: Complete Your Night Time Routine
- Drink 1 glass of water
- Brush your teeth
- Turn off all social media and computers. Power down for the night.
- Pull on fresh pajamas

- If you have a picture book, (or checked one out from the library), lay down in bed and quietly read your book. If you don't have a picture book, listen to a read aloud picture book on YouTube. (There are bunches of videos!)
- Reduce your room lighting to a simple side lamp or fairy lights. Quiet the mind.
- Turn on soft lullaby music or classical music on YouTube

As you begin to feel groggy, turn everything off, snuggle up to your plushie and drift off to sleep. (Make sure to get those 7-8 hours of rest in!).

Day 22: Developing Self-Discipline: Creating an After-Training Plan for Yourself

Welcome to Day 22 of your Little Training! It's hard to believe that we're almost to the end. Today's focus is going to be in creating an after-training plan for yourself to continue your Little space long after you put this book down. The key to self-discipline is recognizing that as a solo Little, you are going to have to be accountable for your own actions. Developing habits now that are desirable to a dominant will aid you in the future. Just as every Little is different, so too is every dominant unique and different. What each dominant is looking for varies, however, there's a general baseline of things a dominant will look for from you. These characteristics include:

- Being joyful and optimistic
- Having emotional maturity
- Being truthful
- Having your personal life in order
- Understanding what you want in a dominant
- Being loyal and understanding
- Being able to switch to Big Me to communicate deeper emotion and issues
- Knowing the fundamental basics of how a D/s relationship operates
- Being open-minded to allowing your dominant to take control and work on you
- Obeying your dominant from a place of love and trust

When you initially connect with your Daddy or Mommy, it's never going to be picture perfect. The deepest D/s relationships are those built over time with tons of experience to develop trust, love, respect and obedience. How does a Little learn to obey and surrender power so freely? The answer is that it begins by developing habits while you're solo to know what you want and what you don't. In order for the Little to be able to trust and love the dominant, they need to love and trust themselves first. For the dominant to be able to work with the Little well, the Little needs to be able to communicate what they're feeling and thinking, what they really like or dislike, what their limits are and what their expectations are from the relationship. In short, you need to know yourself.

Think about some areas that you want to work on within yourself. Only you know what you need to do for personal growth. Part of creating an after-training plan is to develop rules to mould yourself into who you want to be for your future dominant. An example of this would be to create a rule to curb using bad words. Generally speaking, dominants will not approve for Littles to use profanity. As part of your after-training plan, try finding other words to replace these bad words and over time it will become habit.

Today's Challenge: Create a list of after-training rules for yourself in your evening journal reflection and think about areas of yourself in which you want to strive for more personal growth.

After you have completed today's challenge, please move on to complete day 22 tasks.

Day 22 Tasks:

Task #1: Complete Your Morning Routine
- Drink 1 glass of water as soon as you wake up
- Wash your face
- Brush your teeth
- Throw your shower towel into the dryer (if available) and have it tumbling on low-medium heat while you hop into the shower.
- Shower up. While in the shower, think of a song you used to love as a child. Sing that song to yourself as you lather up. Then wrap yourself up in your warm towel afterward. Ahhh...
- Take time to pick out an outfit that is both comfortable, yet makes you feel pretty.
- Put on sunscreen and Chapstick
- Lotion your skin with baby lotion

Task #2: Meditate for 15 minutes

If you have a phone, I want you to download the FREE app. Headspace. It has guided meditation apps that are picked by the program based upon your current mood. If you do not have a phone, go onto YouTube and follow a 15-minute guided meditation video. Allow your breathing to calm and relax your body. Let go of your stresses and fears. Simply be. This daily practice is designed to train you to build up patience in sitting still as you will need to do for your dominant in the future.

Task #3: Browse DDLG/LB Fashion Online

Begin browsing fashion online to formulate your own unique little style! You can also see previous chapters (III., IV., and V. in this book for product and clothing suggestions). There is a style for everyone. Go and find yours!

Task #4: Time to start your normal day, but don't forget your Little snacks!

Whether you're going to school, or staying at home, as you're doing your normal daily schedule I want you to take several breaks throughout the day to refuel with a glass of water and a small snack. These snacks should specifically remind you of Little Me. Some suggestions include: goldfish crackers, animal crackers, cheese cubes, lunchables, cheerios, etc.

Task #5: Stretch those muscles for 20 minutes of exercise!

This act of self-care will keep you feeling good and your body strong. Pick an activity that you already enjoy doing and exercise for 20 minutes.

Task #6: Evening D/s Movie

Every day for the next 25 days I want you to watch a movie that I've hand-picked that is designed to make you think about qualities that dominants should have. Characters in these movies all portray

traits that most dom's exude. Think about the relationship dynamics and then follow up in Task #6 with your evening journal reflection letter.

Tonight's D/s Movie is: *Strictly Ballroom (1992)*

Task #7: Evening Journal Reflection

Now that your day is starting to wind down and you have completed your first D/s movie, I want you to do an evening journal reflection. Instead of a typical diary entry, I want you to write a letter to your future dominant. You can begin by saying: Dear Future Dom... or Dear Dominant... or Dear Daddy/Mommy.... write what feels natural to you. Think about the qualities you want your dominant to have. Write about wishes you hope for, and dates you want to do with them. Write about the movie you watched tonight and things that are going on in your life. This journal will be a special gift to give your dom when you finally come together.

Task #8: Complete Your Night Time Routine

- Drink 1 glass of water
- Brush your teeth
- Turn off all social media and computers. Power down for the night.
- Pull on fresh pajamas
- If you have a picture book, (or checked one out from the library), lay down in bed and quietly read your book. If you don't have a picture book, listen to a read aloud picture book on YouTube. (There are bunches of videos!)
- Reduce your room lighting to a simple side lamp or fairy lights. Quiet the mind.
- Turn on soft lullaby music or classical music on YouTube

As you begin to feel groggy, turn everything off, snuggle up to your plushie and drift off to sleep. (Make sure to get those 7-8 hours of rest in!).

Day 23: The Ideal Dominant: What Are YOU Looking For?

Welcome to Day 23 of your Little Training! Up until this point, I have not yet divulged what characteristics and qualities a dominant should have. On your daily task #6, you have been watching various D/s movies and reflecting upon them. The common thread is that a dominant, specifically a Daddy or Mommy, must possess certain characteristics to make this type of bond thrive. Today we're going to focus on what qualities you should be looking for when choosing a dominant.

- **Patient** – Littles by nature can and will test a dominant's patience. Like a child, a Little wants to try and push her boundaries to see how far she can go. Littles crave attention and can sometimes brat or throw tantrums. In these instances, a dominant must remain patient.
- **A Confidant** – A Little must be able to confide in the dominant any time. He or she must be able to bare their soul to a dominant's sympathetic ear. This is one of the best ways to establish trust within the relationship
- **Protector** – A dominant must be able to impart security to the Little. Littles must be cared for and cherished, like the dominants greatest treasure. Therefore, the dominant must protect the Little for they are precious.
- **Teacher** – A dominant is a teacher to the Little. Like a child, the Little craves to learn and experience new things with their dominant. They need to be able to ask their dominant questions freely because they have a naturally curious mind.
- **Guide** – A dominant must be willing to guide the Little through every aspect of her life. The world is a big, scary, confusing place a lot of times, a Little needs a strong dominant that can guide him or her through it all.
- **Disciplinarian** – This is one of the hardest qualities to sustain as a dominant for their Little because dominants want to nurture and spoil their Little ones. However, it is important for the dominant to realize that he needs to enforce discipline to their Little to preserve their balance of power and to look after their well-being. Littles can and will brat their dominant from time to time. It is in their nature to crave attention.
- **Trustworthy** – Breaking the trust in a D/s relationship is one of the worst things that can happen. A dominant must be trustworthy because it is the most powerful motivator for a Little to submit themselves to the dominant. A Little who fully trusts their dominant is willing to do everything she can to make them happy.
- **Loving** – Finally, a Daddy or Mommy dominant needs to be loving. Littles are very sensitive and fragile. They love hugs and snuggles and lots of loving kisses. The dominant must be able to communicate and express themselves in a clear and firm but loving manner. After all, you catch more flies with honey than vinegar.

Today's Challenge: Think about what qualities you desire in your future dominant. Reflect and make a list in your evening journal letter.

After you've completed this day's challenge, please continue on with your Day 23 tasks.

Day 23 Tasks:

Task #1: Complete Your Morning Routine
- Drink 1 glass of water as soon as you wake up
- Wash your face
- Brush your teeth
- Throw your shower towel into the dryer (if available) and have it tumbling on low-medium heat while you hop into the shower.
- Shower up. While in the shower, think of a song you used to love as a child. Sing that song to yourself as you lather up. Then wrap yourself up in your warm towel afterward. Ahhh...
- Take time to pick out an outfit that is both comfortable, yet makes you feel pretty.
- Put on sunscreen and Chapstick
- Lotion your skin with baby lotion

Task #2: Meditate for 15 minutes
If you have a phone, I want you to download the FREE app. Headspace. It has guided meditation apps that are picked by the program based upon your current mood. If you do not have a phone, go onto YouTube and follow a 15-minute guided meditation video. Allow your breathing to calm and relax your body. Let go of your stresses and fears. Simply be. This daily practice is designed to train you to build up patience in sitting still as you will need to do for your dominant in the future.

Task #3: Browse DDLG/LB Fashion Online
Begin browsing fashion online to formulate your own unique little style! You can also see previous chapters (III., IV., and V. in this book for product and clothing suggestions). There is a style for everyone. Go and find yours!

Task #4: Time to start your normal day, but don't forget your Little snacks!
Whether you're going to school, or staying at home, as you're doing your normal daily schedule I want you to take several breaks throughout the day to refuel with a glass of water and a small snack. These snacks should specifically remind you of Little Me. Some suggestions include: goldfish crackers, animal crackers, cheese cubes, lunchables, cheerios, etc.

Task #5: Stretch those muscles for 20 minutes of exercise!
This act of self-care will keep you feeling good and your body strong. Pick an activity that you already enjoy doing and exercise for 20 minutes.

Task #6: Evening D/s Movie
Every day for the next 25 days I want you to watch a movie that I've hand-picked that is designed to make you think about qualities that dominants should have. Characters in these movies all portray

traits that most dom's exude. Think about the relationship dynamics and then follow up in Task #6 with your evening journal reflection letter.

Tonight's D/s Movie is: *My Fair Lady (1964)*

Task #7: Evening Journal Reflection

Now that your day is starting to wind down and you have completed your first D/s movie, I want you to do an evening journal reflection. Instead of a typical diary entry, I want you to write a letter to your future dominant. You can begin by saying: Dear Future Dom... or Dear Dominant... or Dear Daddy/Mommy.... write what feels natural to you. Think about the qualities you want your dominant to have. Write about wishes you hope for, and dates you want to do with them. Write about the movie you watched tonight and things that are going on in your life. This journal will be a special gift to give your dom when you finally come together.

Task #8: Complete Your Night Time Routine

- Drink 1 glass of water
- Brush your teeth
- Turn off all social media and computers. Power down for the night.
- Pull on fresh pajamas
- If you have a picture book, (or checked one out from the library), lay down in bed and quietly read your book. If you don't have a picture book, listen to a read aloud picture book on YouTube. (There are bunches of videos!)
- Reduce your room lighting to a simple side lamp or fairy lights. Quiet the mind.
- Turn on soft lullaby music or classical music on YouTube

As you begin to feel groggy, turn everything off, snuggle up to your plushie and drift off to sleep. (Make sure to get those 7-8 hours of rest in!).

Day 24: Things Your Future Dominant Should Know About You

Welcome to Day 24 of your Little Training! Generally speaking, in D/s relationships, there is a standard sequence of events that take place prior to the start of a relationship. The dom and sub with communicate and get to know each other. If there is a spark then they will connect and begin to ask questions that target certain aspects that both parties need to know prior to the relationship. Afterwards, a contract a is formed and safe words are put in place. These are the fundamental pieces of a D/s relationship that every Little should be aware of.

Today's lesson, we'll focus on specific areas of information that most dominants will be asking you as they get to know you. Let's delve into each one:

- **Your age** – Most DDLG events and activities require you to be 18+. For the safety of the dom and you, please refrain from entering a D/s relationship until you are a legal adult because this relationship can be sexual in nature.
- **Relationship status** – It is common to find D/s relationships that vary from part-time and full-time. It is important for the Dominant to know of any responsibilities in your personal life like a spouse, children, etc.
- **Living situation** – It is helpful for your Dom to know if you are living at home with your family or a place of your own. Knowing this information will be critical for your dom to create a schedule that works for both of you.
- **Physical attributes** – Your dom wants to know what you look like. Be honest, because just as you are naturally attracted to certain people, your dom is too.
- **Geographic location** – Knowing the general geographic location helps, especially in long distance or online relationships because of time zone differences and scheduling play sessions.
- **Profession** – Divulging whether you are a student or you have a career is another way for your dominant to get to know you better.
- **Health concerns** - If there are any mental health issues, mobility issues, traumas, or health needs that you have – it is vital that you disclose this to your dominant so they can be aware of your needs.
- **Date of last STD test** – Since a lot of D/s relationships can be sexual in nature, it is not uncommon for your dominant to ask when you last took an STD test.
- **Hard and Soft limits** – Part of being a dominant is pushing the Little beyond their comfort zone. However, it is important in the creation of a D/s contract that both hard limits (non-negotiable) and soft limits (negotiable) are declared and upheld.
- **Religious affiliation and/or traditions** – Your dominant needs to know if you have any dietary restrictions (kosher, no pork or beef, halal) or if you have a prayer schedule that needs to be followed.
- **Why you are a Little** – Your dominant needs to know your motivation in entering the relationship. You should be able to tell them why you feel you are a Little.

- **Experience with non-parental spanking** – If you've had experience with spanking in a relationship, this is something you'll want to disclose.
- **Your expectations from a D/l relationship** – Setting expectations is always important to prevent disappointment or misunderstandings.
- **Your best experiences as a Little** – If you have a fond memory in Little space, feel free to share it with your dominant.
- **Your worst experience as a Little** – Likewise, if you've had a negative experience in Little space, you'll need to share that with them as well.
- **Your good and bad triggers** – Everybody has triggers and your dominant needs to know what yours are. These are the things that make you tick or turn you off.
- **Pain threshold** – If physical punishment is something that arouses you, you'll want to discuss how much pain you are comfortable with.
- **Types of pain you enjoy** – Share with your dominant any tools or sex toys you are interested in experiencing together,
- **Preferred punishment method** – Some Littles prefer an over the knee method (otk) so do relay to your dom what punishment method you prefer. See Chapter X for other punishment methods.
- **Nudity comfort level** – Nudity can be a powerful tool that your dom can use during and after training. Shedding your clothes for your dom is symbolic for the Little to shed his or her inhibitions. Once the comfort of clothes is gone, the Little is left vulnerable allowing the dom to establish trust with him or her.
- **Masturbation** – If you engage in self-love practices, your dominant may want control over your orgasms as a form of training. This is something you two should talk about.
- **Communication habits** – You should tell your dominant what kind of communication medium you prefer or most comfortable with (phone, email, chat, Skype, etc.)
- **Your support system** – This is especially important for part time or long distance/online D/s relationships. Since your dominant cannot be there 24/7, they will want to know that you have a support system in place like friends or family that you can rely on if needed.
- **Questions or concerns** – You should take the chance to ask any questions or bring up any concerns you may have. This is the perfect time to do it before you get invested in the relationship. Make sure to note any red flags early on.

Today's Challenge: Create a "stat sheet" and answer these questions to share with your future dominant.

After you're finished with your challenge, please continue on to complete your Day 24 tasks.

<u>**Day 24 Tasks:**</u>

Task #1: Complete Your Morning Routine
- Drink 1 glass of water as soon as you wake up
- Wash your face
- Brush your teeth
- Throw your shower towel into the dryer (if available) and have it tumbling on low-medium heat while you hop into the shower.
- Shower up. While in the shower, think of a song you used to love as a child. Sing that song to yourself as you lather up. Then wrap yourself up in your warm towel afterward. Ahhh...
- Take time to pick out an outfit that is both comfortable, yet makes you feel pretty.
- Put on sunscreen and Chapstick
- Lotion your skin with baby lotion

Task #2: Meditate for 15 minutes
If you have a phone, I want you to download the FREE app. Headspace. It has guided meditation apps that are picked by the program based upon your current mood. If you do not have a phone, go onto YouTube and follow a 15-minute guided meditation video. Allow your breathing to calm and relax your body. Let go of your stresses and fears. Simply be. This daily practice is designed to train you to build up patience in sitting still as you will need to do for your dominant in the future.

Task #3: Browse DDLG/LB Fashion Online
Begin browsing fashion online to formulate your own unique little style! You can also see previous chapters (III., IV., and V. in this book for product and clothing suggestions). There is a style for everyone. Go and find yours!

Task #4: Time to start your normal day, but don't forget your Little snacks!
Whether you're going to school, or staying at home, as you're doing your normal daily schedule I want you to take several breaks throughout the day to refuel with a glass of water and a small snack. These snacks should specifically remind you of Little Me. Some suggestions include: goldfish crackers, animal crackers, cheese cubes, lunchables, cheerios, etc.

Task #5: Stretch those muscles for 20 minutes of exercise!
This act of self-care will keep you feeling good and your body strong. Pick an activity that you already enjoy doing and exercise for 20 minutes.

Task #6: Evening D/s Movie
Every day for the next 25 days I want you to watch a movie that I've hand-picked that is designed to make you think about qualities that dominants should have. Characters in these movies all portray

traits that most dom's exude. Think about the relationship dynamics and then follow up in Task #6 with your evening journal reflection letter.

Tonight's D/s Movie is: *Hart of Dixie (TV Series 2011-2015)*

Task #7: Evening Journal Reflection

Now that your day is starting to wind down and you have completed your first D/s movie, I want you to do an evening journal reflection. Instead of a typical diary entry, I want you to write a letter to your future dominant. You can begin by saying: Dear Future Dom... or Dear Dominant... or Dear Daddy/Mommy.... write what feels natural to you. Think about the qualities you want your dominant to have. Write about wishes you hope for, and dates you want to do with them. Write about the movie you watched tonight and things that are going on in your life. This journal will be a special gift to give your dom when you finally come together.

Task #8: Complete Your Night Time Routine

- Drink 1 glass of water
- Brush your teeth
- Turn off all social media and computers. Power down for the night.
- Pull on fresh pajamas
- If you have a picture book, (or checked one out from the library), lay down in bed and quietly read your book. If you don't have a picture book, listen to a read aloud picture book on YouTube. (There are bunches of videos!)
- Reduce your room lighting to a simple side lamp or fairy lights. Quiet the mind.
- Turn on soft lullaby music or classical music on YouTube

As you begin to feel groggy, turn everything off, snuggle up to your plushie and drift off to sleep. (Make sure to get those 7-8 hours of rest in!).

Day 25: Your Closing Ceremony

Welcome to your final lesson in Little training! By now, you have dedicated nearly one month of your life into learning everything you can about becoming a Little. You have an arsenal of tools to help you navigate your post-training Little lifestyle. You should feel proud of yourself for how far you have come for the past several weeks. I know I'm proud of you!

Today we'll be focusing on wrapping up your training with a simple task that you can hold on to for years to come, picking out the perfect plushie. Every Little has their favorite plushie! Your task today is simple: Go online or to the store and find a stuffed animal or baby blanket that resonates with you. As you shop, you'll know which plushie is the right one because you'll see it and it'll just click. You'll smile and know that that plushie is the one you want to snuggle with every night as you sleep. It's the plushie that you will share with your new Little friends at the next convention or tea party. It will be an important anchor in helping you fall into Little space.

Today's Final Challenge: Go shopping and pick out the perfect plushie!

Now that you've completed your Little training, you possess a deeper understanding of what being a Little is and what the lifestyle is all about. As you meet future dominants, you'll need to take your time to sift through each person in order to find that one dom that feels just right. Below you'll find a questionnaire that you can use to get to know a new dominant. I encourage you to ask these questions in the process of getting to know each other. The more information you can gain, the better clarity you will have in deciding if the relationship is right for you.

25 Questions to Ask A New Dominant

1. How old are you?
2. Where do you live/ What time zone are you in?
3. What do you look like?
4. What's your relationship status?
5. How long have you been a dominant?
6. Do you have any other subs?
7. What are you looking for in a sub?
8. What is your usual style of punishment?
9. Have you ever been a dominant to a Little?
10. Do you expect a part-time or full-time relationship?
11. What do you do for a living?
12. Are you open to creating a contract with me?
13. Do you expect the relationship to be sexual?
14. What are your turn ons? Turn offs?
15. Are there any other kinks you have?
16. Do you intend to meet in person?
17. What are some clothing items you prefer your Little to wear?
18. What was the last D/s relationship you had? And why did it end?
19. What's your motivation for being a Daddy or Mommy?
20. Have you ever attended a DDLG/LB convention before?
21. How do you feel about bratting?
22. When was the last time you took an STD test?
23. What are your pet peeves?
24. Why do you want a relationship with me?
25. Why should I choose you as my Mommy/Daddy?

Chapter XII.

Conclusion & My Story

sat here for quite some time thinking about what to say to you, Dear Reader, about how to end this book. For some of you, it is the start of the journey, and for others the journey has already begun. It is my deepest hope that your path into being a Little is a beautiful one. I wish you many days filled with laughter and love. I hope that you throw out your arms and dance like no one is watching. Let your heart be light and merry, because that is what being a Little is all about. I wish that you will one day make little friends, and together you will make many wonderful, exciting memories. I pray that your future Dominant is kind, generous, humble, and sincere. May you both be filled with deep satisfaction and joy from the bond you will form.

I pray that whatever path you walk, that you walk it with authenticity. Who you are, is unique and special. There is no one quite like you. It doesn't matter if you're a Little boy or girl, tall or short, or if you're thin or curvy. What truly matters is the love you hold in your heart and the happiness you spread in the world. Be you! Be your unique self! March to your own little drum and never let anyone stand in your way. Hold your chin up and remember to not judge anyone whether they are a sexual Little or not, or if they have other kinks or not. We are all ONE community and together we are far more powerful united than divided.

Allow yourself to feel. Your reason for being a Little is special to you. Feel your way through the journey of loving yourself deeper. Nurture your soul with hours and hours of self-care. Your body, mind, and spirit will thank you for it. The ray of sunshine that you are is what your dominant loves about you. Share that light with the world because it needs a whole lot of glitter and sunshine right now. And remember, you're not alone. Starting on the path to DDLG/LB can be a scary one, but you are far from alone. Once upon a time, I was there too. This is my story to becoming a little.

For me, the story begins at Christmas. Why? Because my happiest memories of my childhood were around Christmas time. I remember caroling in the snow, and our whole house being decorated with boughs of evergreen and plaid ribbons. I remember the candles in the window and eating a ham on Christmas Day. It was my favorite time of the year. But life has a funny way of changing things. My childhood became fragmented when my family was torn apart by divorce. Like thousands of others, I grew up bouncing around and by the time I was a "legal adult" I felt utterly lost. Over the course of the years, I lost more than myself. I lost the ability to cope with pain, so I ate. By the time I was in my 20's I was morbidly obese and in need of a lifeline. Eventually I got gastric bypass surgery, and yes, I lost 100 pounds, but I still grappled with finding a sense of identity and making peace with the baggage of my past.

Years later I met a man who became my first Dom. It was a brief relationship that taught me so much. I had no idea that I was a natural submissive. I didn't know anything about DDLG or age regression. Up until that point I had been completely in the dark. Suddenly, it was as if a sheet was pulled off my eyes and I saw people who are just like me! I had found my tribe. For years, I wondered why I had such a playful, silly, happy-go-lucky side of me despite becoming an adult. Through that relationship, I learned to not only accept that part of myself, but to embrace it. I learned what a dominant should act like, and what he shouldn't. Closing that chapter of my life was difficult and filled me with sorrow, but more importantly I was left feeling different. It was as if I couldn't go back to the vanilla world. I knew that even if I never had a Dom again, that I would always want to be involved in the BDSM lifestyle. I knew that I was a Little. Then I connected with my Daddy. It was like slipping on a shoe that just fit.

It took work, patience, and training to come together and bond as deeply as we have. I learned so much about who I am, and who I wish to be. Through my training I was pushed beyond what I thought were my limitations to begin to become to woman I've always hoped to be. He helped me realize that the true love of a dominant isn't when they are snuggled up to you at night, but rather when they are wiping away your tears after you make a giant mistake. It's when they spoon feed you when you're sick, and hold you despite you acting like a giant bag of grumps. He taught me to be thankful, and grateful for having that unconditional love and it has forever changed me. He has forever changed me.

My Daddy is humble, kind, and so patient with my fiery spirit. He guides me to reach goals when I get too scared to try. He pushes me when I feel lazy and begin to procrastinate. He mentors me when I don't understand something, and teaches me something new. And he holds me, because he wants to and because he knows it heals my soul. He is my Daddy, and I am his Little. He is my dominant and to whom I serve with all of my heart.

May all of you find a love within your own D/s relationship that is so powerful and strong that it takes your breath away. May you fall asleep in the warmth of their arms, and wake up spooned and safe. May every part of you be loved, cared for, and cherished. This is my wish for you now and always. Thank you for purchasing this book and giving me your support! I truly hope it has helped you along your path. Cheers, my friend, and may we meet one day at the next Little convention! Xx

Made in the USA
Middletown, DE
15 March 2021